3

# Smart Guide™ to Healing Foods

# About Smart Guides™

Welcome to Smart Guides. Each Smart Guide is created as a written conversation with a learned friend; a skilled and knowledgeable author guides you through the basics of the subject, selecting out the most important points and skipping over anything that's not essential. Along the way, you'll also find smart inside tips and strategies that distinguish this from other books on the topic.

Within each chapter you'll find a number of recurring features to help you find your way through the information and put it to work for you. Here are the user-friendly elements you'll encounter and what they mean:

**The Keys**
Each chapter opens by highlighting in overview style the most important concepts in the pages that follow.

**Smart Move**
Here's where you will learn opinions and recommendations from experts and professionals in the field.

**Street Smarts**
This feature presents smart ways in which people have dealt with related issues and shares their secrets for success.

**Smart Sources**
Each of these sidebars points the way to more and authoritative information on the topic, from organizations, corporations, publications, Web sites, and more.

**Smart Definition**
Terminology and key concepts essential to your mastering the subject matter are clearly explained in this feature.

**F.Y.I.**
Related facts, statistics, and quick points of interest are noted here.

**What Matters, What Doesn't**
Part of learning something new involves distinguishing the most relevant information from conventional wisdom or myth. This feature helps focus your attention on what really matters.

**The Bottom Line**
The conclusion to each chapter, here is where the lessons learned in each section are summarized so you can revisit the most essential information of the text.

One of the main objectives of the *Smart Guide to Healing Foods* is not only to better inform you about which foods are most nutritious but also to make you smarter about the fundamental relationship between eating and health to ensure a lifetime of wellness.

# Smart Guide™ to Healing Foods

Katharine Colton

CADER BOOKS

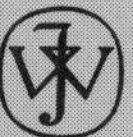

John Wiley & Sons, Inc.

New York • Chichester • Weinheim • Brisbane • Singapore • Toronto

Published by John Wiley & Sons, Inc.
Published simultaneously in Canada



The information contained in this book is not intended to serve as a replacement for professional medical advice. Any use of the information in this book is at the reader's discretion. The author and the publisher specifically disclaim any and all liability arising directly or indirectly from the use or application of any information contained in this book. A health-care professional should be consulted regarding your specific situation.

ISBN 0-471-31860-4

Printed in the United States of America

10 9 8 7 6 5 4 3 2 1

# Contents

# Introduction

The basic tenets of health and healing have been radically revised in recent years. Instead of approaching health from the outside in, we are now approaching it from the inside out, taking care of ourselves so that someone else won't have to. That means adopting a healthy lifestyle and sticking to it every day (or almost every day). Most importantly, it means eating smart and staying active—two small steps that offer gigantic health benefits.

The current dietary wisdom echoes that of our long-ago ancestors, confirming that food is our most potent medicine. Today, scientists are uncovering more and more information about the diverse power of food to prevent and treat everything from headaches to cancer, thanks to an arsenal of ailment-fighting vitamins, minerals, and newly discovered phytonutrients. Much research remains to be done (for example, of the thousands of phytonutrients in your average vegetable, only a few have yet been named and studied), but the crucial connection between food and health has now been validated in study after study, and embraced by even the most cautious of mainstream medical organizations.

The best news is that we have the power to maintain and improve our health with every bite we take. And food is good medicine in more ways than one—unlike other medications, food actually tastes great going down, and enjoyment is an important part of staying healthy.

In the *Smart Guide to Healing Foods* you'll find information on the nutritional benefits of dozens of foods—fruits, vegetables, grains, herbs, and other good things—as well as specific information on which foods are the best medicine for specific ailments. You'll also find flavorful recipes that remind you that smart, healthy eating also tastes great.

Chapter 1 covers the history of healing foods. Chapter 2 looks at the basics of good nutrition. In chapters 3 and 4, you'll find out which foods are the best of the best, offering top nutritional and healing benefits as well as terrific flavor.

Chapter 5 describes healing herbs and spices that add zest as well as nutritional zing to everything you eat. Finally, chapter 6 provides an A to Z of common ailments and the best foods to prevent and treat them.

Remember that food, for all its wonderful health-enhancing and healing properties, is only one type of medicine; it is not a cure for all ills. Many conditions require medical supervision; always consult your health practitioner before embarking on or changing your treatment. And keep in mind that research on the healing benefits of food is still in its preliminary stages. Finally, foods that prove beneficial for one person's arthritis, or migraine, or scratchy throat, or any other malady may do nothing for yours. But eating a diet rich in wholesome, nutrient-rich foods is a surefire bet for improving your overall health—and maybe working some natural healing miracles as well.

So eat up, and eat smart. And here's to your health!

CHAPTER 1

# The Food-Health Connection

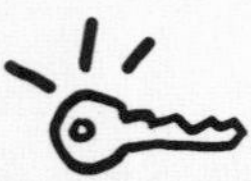

**THE KEYS**

- The ancients knew about food's healing powers—but then science forgot.
- Modern medicine has slowly rediscovered nutrition.
- Plants hold the key to good health.
- The Food Guide Pyramid offers a new architecture for eating well.
- There's more than one way to build a pyramid: you'll discover what alternative diets offer and how to substitute for what they may leave out.

"You are what you eat." Today that phrase may seem as obvious as "the earth is round," but at times both have their share of skeptics. This chapter looks at the food-health connection from its earliest days to the present, from ages-old traditions to cutting-edge scientific research.

# The History of Healing Foods

Our earliest ancestors subsisted on a plant-rich diet, occasionally supplemented by meat or fish. No one thought of this regime as "healthy"; it was simply a matter of necessity. McDonald's was not an option. Starvation, however, was a very real possibility, and it led people to try eating almost anything they could get their hands on or spears into.

So, too, with the early use of plants as medicine; necessity drove early peoples to experiment with herbs, seeds, fruits, and vegetables to treat ailments. They carefully observed and remembered which foods were effective and passed this information on from generation to generation. For example:

- The ancient Egyptians treated infections, headaches, and other ailments with garlic; a document from 1500 B.C. includes more than two hundred prescriptions using garlic!

- Ancient Greeks and Romans used apples to treat congestion, fever, flu, and other illnesses.

• For centuries the Chinese have used ginger to treat nausea.

Despite myriad changes in culture, habits, and lifestyle, the discoveries made by ancient cultures continued to have an impact on both eating and health habits throughout the centuries. Take the phrase "An apple a day keeps the doctor away." Based on the ancient Greek saying "To eat an apple going to bed, will make a doctor beg his bread," it has survived to this day.

Yet did you ever stop to think about the validity of this aphorism? If not, you're not alone.

**F.Y.I.**

Hippocrates, known as the father of modern medicine, put it succinctly way back in 400 B.C.: "Let food be your medicine and medicine be your food."

## The Price of Progress

Somewhere around the middle of the twentieth century, Americans lost sight of the connection between food and health, between what we eat and what we are. "Progress"—cutting-edge research, high-tech medical equipment, and a fleet of new pharmaceuticals—brought an obsession with the latest, fastest, most modern treatments. Physicians fell in love with new "miracle drugs" such as antibiotics; many started believing that pharmaceuticals were the only legitimate treatment for any ailment.

The role of diet suddenly became irrelevant. Obsessed by the shiniest, newest methods of detecting and treating disease, physicians lost sight of the roots of illness—and of good health.

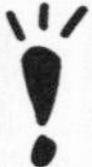

**SMART MOVE**

Back in the 1950s, when the medical establishment was enthralled by pharmaceuticals and high-tech equipment, nutritionist Adelle Davis was insisting that diet was a direct cause of many diseases. The author of *Let's Eat Right to Keep Fit* (1954), among many other titles, Davis considered the prevailing approach to wellness completely backward in its focus on cures rather than causes. "Thousands upon thousands of persons have studied disease," she wrote. "Almost no one has studied health." At the time, she was dismissed as a quack.

## Faster, Not Better

At the same time, our increasingly high-speed, modernized society fell in love with fast food, and burgers and fries replaced many a three-square meal. Fresh fruits and vegetables—along with the vitamins they contain—nearly disappeared from the dinner table, and from public consciousness.

Our diet changed—and continues to change—more during this period than during the thousands of years preceding it. Unfortunately, while these changes brought *more* choices to our table, they did not bring *healthier* choices.

## The Big Question

In the 1970s, a few researchers finally began asking why, when so much money and research and brain power were being channeled toward health care, wasn't there a decline in the rates of cancer, heart disease, and other illnesses?

Around this time, some really puzzling data came to light: many less wealthy and less technologically savvy countries had lower rates of heart disease and cancer than the United States. At that point researchers realized they had to start looking at other factors, such as eating habits and lifestyle.

They discovered that in less developed countries, diets consisted mostly of basic, unrefined foods such as fruits, vegetables, and grains. This contrasted sharply with the prevailing diet in the United States and other wealthy countries: meat and potatoes, fast food, and a paltry amount of fresh fruits and vegetables.

## The Simple Answer

Although some researchers were reluctant to acknowledge it, the evidence pointed to a direct link between diet and health. The diets that seemed to offer protection from disease were those that were low in fat and high in fiber, fruits, and vegetables. The American diet is just the opposite—high in fat and low in fiber and plant foods. Therefore, a high-fat, low-fiber diet must increase the chances of developing certain diseases, such as heart disease and cancer, since those diseases are so prevalent in the United States.

## Secret Ingredients

Once the diet-health connection was (re)established, scientists began to ask another question. Why did a diet low in fat and rich in fiber and plant foods offer more protection against disease?

They theorized that some ingredients in this diet's main component—plant foods—might play a protective role. So researchers began analyzing fruits and vegetables to try to find these ingredients. They found that plant foods are loaded with vitamins, including beta-carotene (the plant form of vitamin A), C, and E, as well as minerals such as potassium and selenium. They also discovered that fruits and vegetables contain many other chemical compounds, now known as phytonutrients, that scientists had never before detected.

Researchers then looked for links between these substances and diseases such as cancer and heart disease. Sure enough, they found that people who ate diets low in those vitamins and miner-

**SMART DEFINITION**

**Antioxidants**

Nutrients that help protect against disease and strengthen the body's immune system. Among other functions, antioxidants promote tissue repair and prevent the formation of harmful molecules—known as free radicals—that can trigger cancer.

als had a much higher risk of disease. They also found evidence that many of those newly discovered phytonutrients were at least as important in protecting our bodies as vitamins and minerals—if not more so.

## Coming Full Circle

Since then, research has not only validated the simple credo "you are what you eat" but has also unearthed an incredible array of healing properties in foods, reopening our eyes to the traditional concept of food as medicine.

Among the findings:

• Certain compounds in onions and garlic can discourage blood clotting and increase cancer resistance.

• Beta-carotene and vitamins C and E, found in many fruits and vegetables, act as antioxidants, helping the body to defend against disease, thus slowing the aging process.

• Pectin, the type of fiber found in apples, helps lower cholesterol levels and may protect against diabetes.

Ironically, technology—which distracted scientists from the food-health connection in the first place—has now made it possible to detect previously unknown compounds and chemical processes and observe their effects in the body.

Today, even notoriously cautious and conservative scientific groups agree that nutrition is an essential part of disease prevention and treatment, and that nutritional deficiencies may be the cause of many problems that previously baffled physicians.

## From Proof to Practice

Now that studies have proved what our ancestors knew all along—that food is a crucial component of health and healing—what are we doing about it? Not as much as we should, for the most part. Many people in this land of plenty seem determined to eat whatever they please, taking to heart Mark Twain's adage: "Part of the secret of success in life is to eat what you like and let the food fight it out inside." In fact, that's more like a recipe for disaster.

If—as truckloads of evidence proves—diet can help protect against such illnesses as cancer and heart disease, then we must be doing something wrong considering that these diseases are still our nation's top killers.

## The Push for a Healthier Diet

Americans' not-so-good (or downright lousy) eating habits can't be blamed on lack of information.

After the initial research linking diet and disease, major health organizations such as the National Cancer Institute, the American Heart Association, and the National Academy of Science, as well as universities around the world, launched new programs devoted to researching the role of dietary changes in preventing illness. Among their findings:

**F.Y.I.**

According to the Cancer Research Foundation of America, about 35 percent of cancer is caused by choosing the wrong foods too often. (And many experts think this figure is too low.)

• National Cancer Institute research showed that people who eat five or more daily servings of fruits and vegetables may reduce their risk of prostate, bladder, esophagus, stomach, and possibly other cancers.

• The National Heart and Lung Institute found that eating omega-3 fatty acids (found in salmon, mackerel, and other fatty fish) may reduce the risk of cardiovascular disease in men by as much as 40 percent. (Women have not yet been studied.)

• The Framingham Children's Study found that children with the highest intake of calcium-rich foods had the lowest blood pressure. Similar studies on adults have shown the same results.

• Researchers at New York Medical College found that eating one-half to one clove of garlic a day lowered cholesterol levels by about 9 percent.

## The Food Guide Pyramid

The most high-profile response to the new findings came from the United States Department of Agriculture (USDA), which revised its nutritional guidelines to reflect the new research. The old guidelines, established back in the 1950s, consisted of a pie cut into four equal pieces, with each representing one of four food groups: meat, dairy, grains, and fruits and vegetables. The simple message: eat a generous portion of each every day.

Replacing the outdated pie is the new USDA Food Guide Pyramid, which apportions foods quite differently.

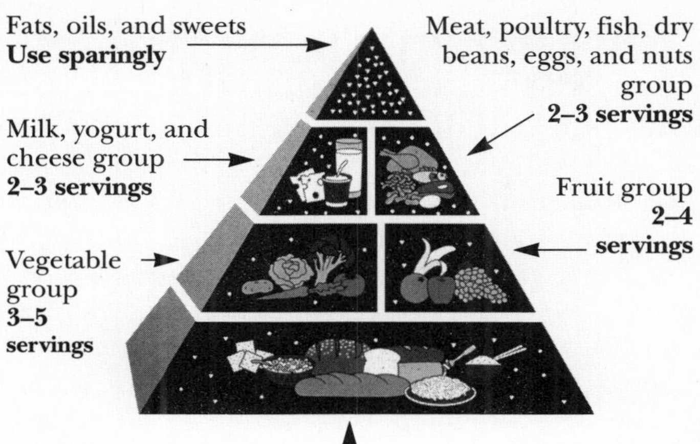


*Source:* U.S. Department of Agriculture

Instead of the traditional four food groups, the pyramid has five, and they no longer get equal billing. The goal is to eat from the bottom on up:

The base of the pyramid is dedicated to those fiber- and nutrient-rich foods found most effective in maintaining health and fighting illness. The USDA advises choosing most of your calories from foods in the grain group (6 to 11 servings), the vegetable group (3 to 5 servings), and the fruit group (2 to 4 servings).

As you go up the pyramid, the recommended serving sizes go down. More moderate servings of dairy foods (2 to 3 servings) and meat and beans (2 to 3 servings) reflect recent findings on protein requirements and the potential dangers of dietary fat and cholesterol.

At the top of the pyramid is a new group: fats, oils, and sweets. The USDA recommends eating these "sparingly," again reflecting research linking fat intake to heart disease and other health problems.

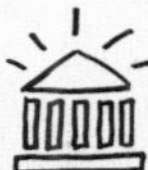

**SMART SOURCES**

These two books offer an abundance of information about healthy eating:

*The Nutrition Bible*
by Barbara Deskins and Jean E. Anderson

*The American Dietetic Association's Complete Food & Nutrition Guide*
by Roberta Larson Duyff

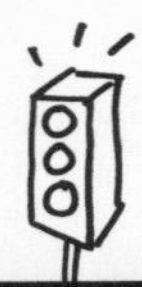

**WHAT MATTERS, WHAT DOESN'T**

**What Matters**

- Eating at least five servings of fruits and vegetables a day.
- Choosing whole-grain, fiber-rich complex carbohydrates to meet your grain quota.
- Avoiding excess fat.

**What Doesn't**

- Rigidly adhering to the USDA's food guide pyramid; healthy alternatives are offered by the Asian, Mediterranean, and vegetarian pyramids.

# Other Pyramid Schemes

When U.S. researchers began examining the diets of other countries with lower rates of heart disease and cancer, they helped instigate a new, more global approach to eating. Americans paid attention to the news that people in Asian and Mediterranean countries were living longer, healthier lives. As a result, there's been a gradual shift toward new foods and new ways of cooking. It's no longer heresy to admit that our way of eating isn't necessarily the best way.

At the same time, many people began experimenting with vegetarianism—either going whole hog (so to speak) or incorporating aspects of vegetarian cooking into their diets. Avoiding meat became not just a political choice but a health choice.

Alternative diets now have their own food pyramids, which share some traits with the USDA's version, but diverge in important ways. The main difference is that these alternative plans limit consumption of meat or dairy, or both, to a few times a month—or not at all. Instead, they emphasize legumes, nuts, and (except for the vegetarian pyramid) fish, all foods proved to pack a disease-fighting wallop. And both the Asian and vegetarian pyramids incorporate daily exercise.

All the pyramids work from bottom to top: you should choose most of your foods from the base and eat less as you near the peak.

## The Asian Way

**Advantages of the Asian Food Plan**

• Fish, nuts, seeds, and beans (including super-healthy soybeans and soy products) are the main protein source, rather than dairy or meat, which

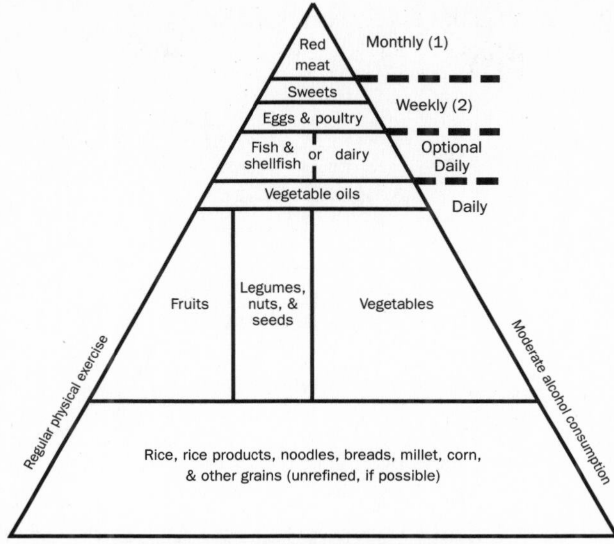


*Adapted from "The Traditional Healthy Asian Diet Pyramid"*


means this diet is very low in fat. Studies show that people who eat little or no meat have much lower rates of heart disease, diabetes, gallstones, high blood pressure, and stroke.

• Large amounts of fruit, vegetables, and grains provide lots of fiber; in fact, the Chinese get 33 grams of fiber each day compared to the average American intake of 11 to 12 grams (the USDA recommends 25 grams).

• Regular exercise is an integral part of the plan.

**Disadvantages**

Because the Asian plan has little dairy, it is low in fat; the down side is that it's also low in calcium. If you follow this plan, you're best off supplementing it with low-fat dairy foods.

## The Mediterranean Way

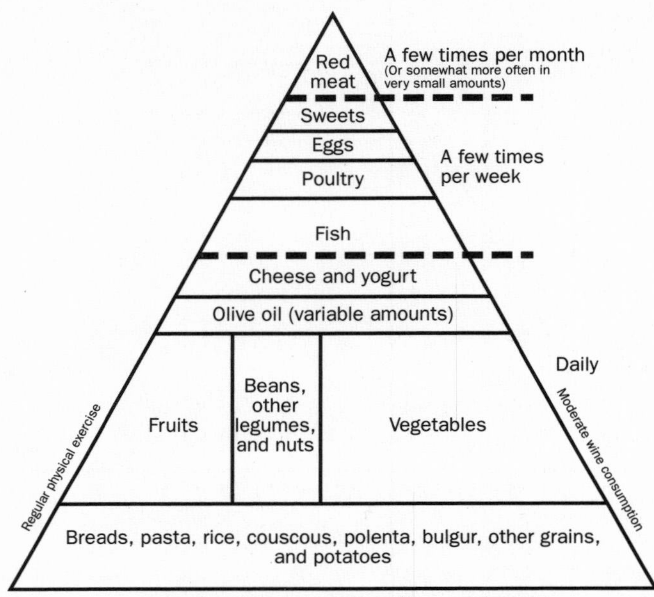


*Adapted from "The Traditional Healthy Mediterranean Diet Pyramid"*
*Copyright © 1994 by Oldways Preservation & Exchange Trust*

The Mediterranean food plan is based on the traditional diets of southern Europe.

**Advantages of the Mediterranean Food Plan**

• Low-fat fish, nuts, beans, and other legumes are the main protein sources; meats are generally eaten only a few times a month.

• Large amounts of fruit, vegetables, and whole grains provide plenty of fiber.

• Olive oil is the healthiest type of fat you can consume; it also contains heart-protecting compounds.

• Studies show that moderate amounts of red wine are good for your heart.

• Regular exercise is an integral part of the plan.

**Disadvantages**
The Mediterranean diet is nearly 40 percent fat. (Most American health organizations recommend 25 to 30 percent, tops.) Still, that doesn't seem to hurt the Mediterraneans any.

## The Vegetarian Way

Vegetarian diets vary widely; the pyramid represents the most common eating habits of vegetarians around the world.

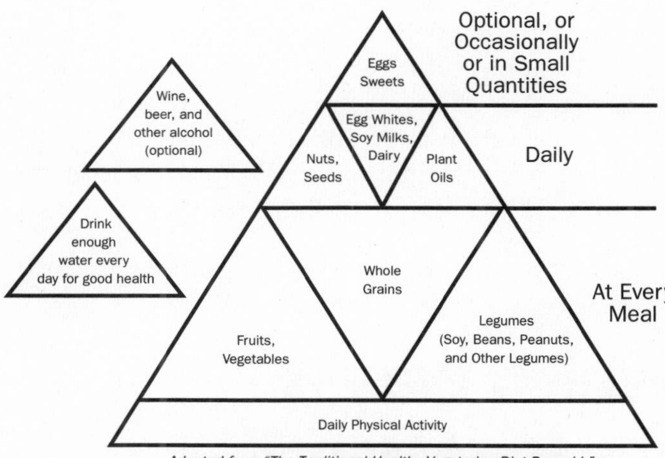


*Adapted from "The Traditional Healthy Vegetarian Diet Pyramid," Copyright © 1997 Oldways Preservation & Exchange Trust*

**Advantages of the Vegetarian Food Plan**
• Instead of meat, plant foods—including soy, beans, and other legumes—are combined with whole grains to provide protein. As noted earlier, studies show that people who eat little or no meat are at much lower risk of developing many serious health problems.

**SMART SOURCES**

The following organizations offer information-filled Web sites and brochures on nutrition:

International Food Information Council
1100 Connecticut Ave. NW, Suite 430
Washington, D.C. 20036
202-296-6540
www.ificinfo.health.org

Request: *10 Tips to Healthy Eating* and *The Food Guide Pyramid: Your Personal Guide to Healthful Eating.*

United States Dept. of Agriculture
Center for Nutrition Policy and Promotion
1120 20th St. NW, Suite 200
Washington, D.C. 20036
202/418-2312
www.usda.gov/fcs/cnnp

Request: *Dietary Guidelines for Americans.* Go to the USDA's Consumer Information Center: http://www.pueblo.gsa.gov

• Because of the high proportion of plant foods in this diet, vegetarians eat, on average, three times as much dietary fiber as the average American.

• Vegetarians get most of their fat from heart-healthy sources such as nuts, seeds, and plant oils; they also consume, on average, less fat than non-vegetarians.

• Regular exercise is an integral part of the daily plan.

**Disadvantages**
None, as long as you choose your foods wisely. Be sure to get your daily protein quotient by eating enough grains and legumes. Vegetarians also have to be careful about getting enough vitamin $B_{12}$, which the body uses to make red blood cells. It's found naturally only in animal foods, but you can get enough by eating fortified foods such as cereals and soy milk.

## Which Way Is the Best Way?

As scientists continue to learn about food's powerful effects on the body, new information will trickle down to the USDA and other health organizations, and they'll revise their nutritional guidelines accordingly. For now, there's no nutritional formula that can guarantee optimal health. But if you use any of the food pyramids as a basic guide, you're guaranteed to get a wide array of the nutrients—both known and yet-to-be-discovered—essential to your good health.

*A caveat:* The food guide pyramid and its variants are designed to meet the needs of basically healthy individuals. If you have a disease or other ailment, the best foods for you may be very different from those in the food pyramids, depending on the type of treatment you are receiving or how you feel. Your health practitioner can advise you about the best diet for your special needs; also see chapter 6 for a rundown of foods that have been found to be beneficial for specific health problems.

Some scientists predict that foods will soon be specially designed and prescribed, just like drugs, and used in very specific combinations to achieve some new state of über-health. But in the meantime, what's most important to your health is eating a wide variety of low-fat, nutritious foods; maintaining a good balance of fats, proteins, and carbohydrates to keep you energized; and making sure you eat a minimum of five fruits and vegetables each day to ensure that you get plenty of fiber, vitamins, minerals, and other micronutrients. (If you need some incentive to shape up your diet, read on: chapter 2 explains just what these nutrients do for you.)

In the chapters ahead you will learn not only which foods are best for keeping all your parts in top working condition, but also which foods are the best prescription to fight specific health problems—so you can become your own personal food physician.

**THE BOTTOM LINE**

The thoughts that food can promote health and healing is no longer just folklore; researchers have validated many ancient practices with hard facts. With more and more findings about the effects of food on health and disease, it's clear that some of the best medicine is not in a bottle but on your plate.

CHAPTER 2

# The Healing Nutrients

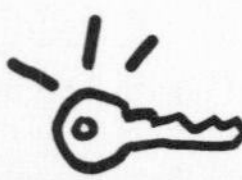

**THE KEYS**

- Everybody needs fat, protein, and carbohydrate, and you'll learn how much and what kind of each are best for you.
- Vitamins and minerals are crucial: here's what they do and where to find them.
- Do you need a pill to get your fill of the RDAs?
- Your body can't survive—and thrive—without fiber and water.
- Phytonutrients are little chemicals that pack a big punch.

You can pay a nutritionist to tell you what to eat (some will even come clean out your refrigerator for you), or you can buy the latest best-selling "breakthrough supernutrition diet" that promises to help you achieve immortality. But while it's eminently wise to discuss your particular health needs with a qualified practitioner, there's only one person who can ensure that you eat right on a daily basis: you.

To be your own nutritionist, you need to educate yourself about food. When you understand what your body needs to keep energized, healthy, and strong, and which nutritional components make this happen, you'll be empowered to make your own smart food choices. This chapter aims to help you reach that goal.

## The Macronutrients: Fat, Protein, and Carbohydrates

Macronutrients are the components in food that give your body energy. Fat, protein, and carbohydrates are all essential to your body in different ways, and you need the right balance of each to maintain optimum health.

There's an ongoing argument—carried out vociferously on bookstore shelves—about what constitutes the "right balance." High-protein and high-carbohydrate diets go in and out of fashion; at various times each has been touted as the key to fitness and health. But fads aside, every major health organization recommends the same ratio of fat, protein, and carbohydrates, the formula that's been found to provide your body with a balanced daily dose of energy and nutrients.

Unless you have a disease or other ailment that requires a different balance of nutrients, you will benefit most by learning about the healthiest fat, protein, and carbohydrate choices, not by seeking some new dietary formula.

**SMART DEFINITION**

**Calorie**

A unit of energy contained in food. Four components in food provide calories:

- fat—provides 9 calories per gram
- protein—provides 4 calories per gram
- carbohydrate—provides 4 calories per gram
- alcohol—provides 7 calories per gram

## Fat: The Maligned Nutrient

Fat is the most concentrated form of energy you can consume. It provides more than twice as many calories per gram than protein or carbohydrates.

Although you don't need much fat in your diet, you do need some. Besides giving you energy, fat supplies essential fatty acids and enables your body to store the fat-soluble vitamins A, D, E, and K. Thanks to those essential fatty acids, your hair and skin don't dry out, you sleep at night, and a healthy mood is maintained.

### The Trouble with Fat

Amidst the barrage of health advice, the message that's come through loudest and clearest is that fat is bad for you. It makes you gain weight, it causes all sorts of diseases, and it is to be shunned. No wonder that in survey after survey, consumers consistently rate fat their top nutrition concern.

But like so much popular nutritional "wisdom," that's a vast simplification of a complex topic. You have already learned about the good things fat does for your body. And while fat's bad rap is grounded in fact, a lot of fat-related health hazards

**SMART DEFINITION**

**Essential fatty acids**

Two polyunsaturated fats, linoleic acid and linolenic acid, are needed to keep the body functioning. They're found in leafy green vegetables, walnuts, sunflower seeds, and canola, corn, cottonseed, safflower, soybean, sunflower, and walnut oils.

can be averted by choosing the right kinds of fat rather than eliminating it altogether.

One problem is that because fat tastes so good it's tempting to eat way more than you should. Your body quickly takes any excess fat and stores it as body fat, which can lead to obesity, and in turn to diabetes, high blood pressure, heart disease, stroke, and certain cancers.

Even if you've got a terrific metabolism and don't gain an ounce from fatty foods, a high-fat diet can still be deadly. The fats found in meats, snack foods, and fatty dairy products clog the arteries of thin as well as heavy people, and put everyone at risk for disease.

## The Right—and Wrong—Kinds of Fat

Some fats do your body good; others do just the opposite. The difference comes down to fatty acids—the basic chemical units in fat. Fatty acids are molecules made up mostly of carbon and hydrogen. The more hydrogen they contain, the more saturated they are. Saturated fats contain the most hydrogen; polyunsaturated fats contain the least.

### The Fats to Avoid

Saturated fat is found in meat, high-fat dairy foods, tropical oils (such as coconut oil and palm kernel oil), and hydrogenated (solidified) vegetable oils. You should strive to minimize this type of fat because it promotes the formation of cholesterol in the body, and therefore is linked to cardiovascular disease.

Scientists have recently targeted another kind of

bad fat, called "trans" fat, which acts like saturated fat in the body. Trans fat, which makes up 5 to 10 percent of the fat content in American diets, is a "hybrid" fat made by adding hydrogen atoms to a polyunsaturated fat to make it more saturated. Listed on food labels as hydrogenated or partially hydrogenated fat, it's found in most margarine, commercial baked goods, and deep-fried foods that use hardened vegetable oils.

Like saturated fat, trans fat should be avoided because it promotes the formation of cholesterol in the body.

### The Fats to Enjoy—in Moderation

Unsaturated fats include monounsaturated fat and polyunsaturated fat. Monounsaturated fats are found in olive, peanut, and canola oils. Polyunsaturated fats are found in most other plant oils, including safflower, soybean, corn, sunflower, sesame, and cottonseed oils; fish oil; and oil from nuts, such as walnuts, hazelnuts, pecans, almonds, and peanuts.

Unsaturated fat is the kind you should eat because it's a great energy source, it contains essential fatty acids, and it actually *lowers* blood cholesterol levels.

## How Much Fat Should You Eat?

In terms of your heart's health, the amount of trans fat and saturated fat you consume is more important than the total amount of fat in your diet. Health experts recommend substituting healthy unsaturated

**F.Y.I.**

About 18 grams of saturated fat per day is a reasonable amount to strive for (that means strive for no more; less is fine!).

fats (monounsaturated and polyunsaturated) for the bad kind—for example, using natural vegetable oils in cooking.

Still, most health experts recommend limiting fat to no more than 30 percent of total daily calories. Some prefer 20 percent, with less than 10 percent of calories coming from saturated fat.

If you eat a healthy diet consisting mostly of fresh fruits, vegetables, and whole grains, along with low-fat proteins, you probably don't need to monitor your fat intake; you're doing fine. But if you eat a fair amount of packaged foods and added fat, you should figure out your daily fat intake by reading nutrition labels on the foods you use. These labels are based on a 2,000-calorie diet; so if you eat 2,000 calories a day, you'd figure:

calories from fat should be no more than 600
(2,000 x .30 = 600)

or no more than about 67 grams fat
(600 calories ÷ 9 calories per gram
of fat = 67).

If you're aiming for 20 percent of your calories from fat, that would come out to 400 calories, or no more than about 44 grams of fat.

**Recommended upper limits of total fat and saturated fat intake at different calorie levels:**

1,200—total fat 40 grams, saturated fat 16 grams

1,600—total fat 53 grams, saturated fat 18 grams

2,000—total fat 65 grams, saturated fat 20 grams

2,500—total fat 80 grams, saturated 25 grams

## The Perils of Cholesterol

Cholesterol is a fatlike substance manufactured by your body and also found in animal foods high in saturated fat such as: egg yolks, meat, poultry, fish, and high-fat milk products.

Since you've no doubt heard that cholesterol is linked to serious diseases, the obvious question is: why does your body make it? Like fat, cholesterol is essential for various physical functions: it's an important part of cell membranes and a building block for important hormones. Your body makes *at least* enough cholesterol to fulfill these functions; some people manufacture more than they need and have naturally elevated blood cholesterol levels.

Excess cholesterol, whether manufactured by your body or provided by a diet high in saturated fat and cholesterol, can clog the arteries, leading to heart attack or stroke.

That's why you should monitor your cholesterol level. When you ask your doctor to measure it for you, make sure you find out not only your overall cholesterol level but also the ratio of "bad" and "good" cholesterol. Low-density lipoprotein (LDL) is the bad kind, the one that sticks to your artery walls. High-density lipoprotein (HDL) is the good kind; it transports dangerous cholesterol out of the blood and into the liver for disposal. Ideally, you want your HDL to be higher than your LDL. The National Cholesterol Education Program recommends keeping your total cholesterol below 200; LDL should be below 130, and HDL above 65.

### Keeping Cholesterol in Check

Most people can keep cholesterol under control by getting plenty of exercise and eating a diet rich

**F.Y.I.**

Saturated fats raise cholesterol levels more than dietary cholesterol does. For example, eating shrimp, which are high in cholesterol but contain unsaturated fat, is better for you than eating so-called "cholesterol-free" cookies, which are likely to be laden with saturated or hydrogenated fats. So check nutrition labels for saturated fat rather than those "cholesterol-free" claims.

in high-fiber foods. (You'll learn more about the benefits of fiber later in this chapter.) Concentrate on unprocessed foods such as whole grains, fruits, and vegetables.

You don't need to go so far as to eliminate all high-cholesterol foods from your diet; many of them are also high in essential nutrients. You're better off watching out for cholesterol-raising saturated fats, which are found in many—but not all—of the same foods.

## Protein Facts

Protein provides your body with nine essential amino acids, chemical compounds that serve as the building blocks, repairers, and regenerators of muscle and tissue, necessary for a strong, healthy body. Your body contains anywhere from 10,000 to 50,000 kinds of protein; everything from hair to skin to blood to enzymes and hormones is made of the stuff. But beware of those who tell you that you can't get enough protein in your diet: consuming more than your body needs is not only unnecessary but potentially harmful.

### How Much Do You Need?

It's essential to consume protein daily because your body cannot store it the way it stores fats. It's pretty easy to get enough in a basic, well-balanced diet, and in fact most Americans already consume more than enough. Nutritionists generally warn against eating more than the Recommended Daily Allowance—50 grams for women over twenty-five, and 63 grams for men over twenty-five—because many protein-rich foods are high in fat, and high-protein diets are hard for your kidneys to process and may damage them.

## Complete versus Incomplete Proteins

Complete proteins (also known as animal proteins) contain all the amino acids you need, in the amounts you need, to stay healthy. They are found in foods such as eggs, meat, fish, poultry, milk and other dairy products.

Incomplete proteins (also known as vegetable proteins) lack one or more essential amino acids. The following plant foods are good sources of incomplete protein: legumes, including peanuts, dried beans, peas, and soybeans; grains, especially whole grains; and potatoes.

Vegetarians combine incomplete proteins, such as beans and brown rice, in order to form complete proteins and get all the essential amino acids.

## The Energizers: Carbohydrates

Carbohydrates are the sugars and starches that provide most of your body fuel and keep your central nervous system, and thus your brain, in

### Recommended Daily Protein Intake

| Age | Weight | Protein Needed |
|---|---|---|
| **Children** | | |
| 1 to 3 yrs. | 29 lbs. | 16 g. |
| 4 to 6 yrs. | 44 lbs. | 24 g. |
| 7 to 10 yrs. | 62 lbs. | 28 g. |
| **Men and boys** | | |
| 11 to 14yrs. | 99 lbs. | 45 g. |
| 15 to 18 yrs. | 145 lbs. | 59 g. |
| 19 to 24 yrs. | 160 lbs. | 59 g. |
| 25 to 50 yrs. | 174 lbs. | 63 g. |
| 51+ yrs. | 170 lbs. | 63 g. |
| **Women and girls** | | |
| 11 to 14 yrs. | 101 lbs. | 46 g. |
| 15 to 18 yrs. | 120 lbs. | 44 g. |
| 19 to 24 yrs. | 128 lbs. | 46 g. |
| 25 to 50 yrs. | 138 lbs. | 50 g. |
| 51+ yrs. | 140 lbs. | 50 g. |
| **Pregnant women** | | 60 g. |
| **Nursing mothers** | | |
| First 6 months | | 65 g. |
| Second 6 months | | 65 g. |

**F.Y.I.**

There's no health benefit to eating brown sugar instead of white. But honey's another story. Though it can also cause tooth decay and is almost as caloric as sugar, honey does have health advantages: it helps fight bacteria and may offer other therapeutic benefits.

working order. In other words, they're crucial. That's why most nutrition experts recommend getting about 60 percent of your daily calories from carbohydrates.

When carbohydrates enter your body, they break down into a simple sugar called glucose. Glucose enters your bloodstream and supplies you with physical and mental energy; it is also stored as glycogen in the liver and muscle tissue, to provide energy reserves. Because your body constantly needs its glycogen stores replenished—particularly if you are active—carbohydrate calories are more likely to be used as glycogen than converted to body fat. That means—despite all the fad diet books that will tell you otherwise—a diet rich in carbohydrates can help you maintain a healthy weight. And that's crucial to your overall health.

The key is to eat complex, not simple, carbohydrates. Simple carbohydrates are found in sugar and other sweeteners, as well as colas, fruit juices, desserts, and other sweet foods. They are easily converted to glucose and are quickly absorbed into your blood, giving you a jolt of energy.

• Complex carbohydrates are found in grains, potatoes, root and starchy vegetables, and dried peas and beans. Because they are made up of hundreds or thousands of glucose molecules, they break down more slowly in the body, especially if the foods that contain them also contain fiber. This makes complex carbohydrates an excellent source of slow-burning energy.

## Sugar: Friend or Foe?

Sugar isn't just the white stuff you spoon onto your shredded wheat. Sugar also occurs naturally in the body during carbohydrate breakdown, and it's a component of many nutritious foods such as milk, fruits, vegetables, cereals, breads, and grains.

Even if you wanted to, you probably couldn't eliminate all sugars from your diet. Nor should you try. Sugar, despite its bad reputation, is not innately bad for you. Although you should monitor your intake of sugar—as well as other empty calories—to avoid weight gain, you don't need to eliminate it for the sake of good health. A little sugar can be good for the soul.

And despite much suspicion to the contrary, scientific evidence indicates that sugar does *not* cause any of the following: hyperactivity, criminal behavior, diabetes, heart disease, acne, or obesity (although sugar can contribute, fatty foods are the main cause).

But sugar *does* cause tooth decay—so be sure to brush thoroughly after eating sugary foods.

# The Micronutrients

Fat, protein, and carbohydrates play the most tangible role in your body, providing the energy that keeps you moving. But it's the behind-the-scenes players—vitamins, minerals, phytonutrients, fiber, and water—that enable your body to turn those nutrients into energy and function effectively and smoothly in your body; and that's just one of the myriad functions they serve. Researchers are learning more every day about what these noncaloric nutrients do for your health.

# Vital Vitamins

There are 13 known vitamins—organic compounds that are required to keep the body healthy and free of disease. Some, such as A, D, and E, are fat-soluble and can damage the liver if consumed in excess amounts; others, such as C, are water-soluble, and excess amounts of them will be flushed out of the body. The following list tells you what each vitamin does for your body, how much of each you should consume, and the best food sources for each. You'll learn more about the top nutrient-packed foods in later chapters.

## Vitamin A

**What it does:** promotes growth of cells and tissue repair, maintains healthy skin; aids in night and color vision; and boosts the immune system. Its precursor, beta-carotene, is an antioxidant.
**What it may do:** prevent premature aging of the skin; as Retin-A, it is commonly used to treat wrinkles. It may also prevent cataracts among the elderly; a recent study found that women who ate foods rich in beta-carotene had a 39 percent lower risk of developing cataracts. Several studies show a link between beta-carotene intake and reduced risk of heart disease and stroke. And beta-carotene and vitamin A may provide strong protection against many forms of cancer, including cancers of the stomach, colon, mouth, throat, esophagus, bladder, cervix, lungs, and breasts.
**RDA:** 5,000 IUs (international units). *Warning:* because vitamin A can be toxic in high doses, you should not consume more than 25,000 IUs per day unless under supervised care.

**Where to find it:** carrots, sweet potatoes, tomatoes, mangoes, cantaloupe, dried apricots, and other red, yellow, and orange fruits and vegetables; leafy green vegetables; liver; whole milk; eggs; cheese; fatty fish.

## Vitamin $B_1$—Thiamin

**What it does:** converts carbohydrates, alcohol, and fats into energy; regulates function of the heart, muscles, nerves, and digestive system.
**What it may do:** reduce risk of cataracts; improve physical and mental well-being by stimulating the nervous system.
**RDA:** 1.5 milligrams.
**Where to find it:** wheat germ, peanuts, sunflower seeds, oatmeal, enriched cereal, whole-grain bread, corn, melon, liver, and pork.

## Vitamin $B_2$—Riboflavin

**What it does:** produces energy from food, promotes growth in children, maintains healthy skin and mucous membranes.
**What it may do:** help the body handle physical stress from exercise and other causes; detoxify chemicals in alcohol and tobacco that may cause esophageal cancer.
**RDA:** 1.7 milligrams.
**Where to find it:** milk (packaged so that it's not exposed to light), yogurt, eggs, cheese, meat, oily fish, crab, mussels, enriched cereals, mushrooms, almonds, and pumpkin seeds.

## Vitamin $B_3$—Niacin

**What it does:** produces energy from food, maintains digestive and reproductive systems, pro-

## Do You Need Supplements?

Lots of people operate under the illusion that as long as they pop a daily multivitamin, they needn't bother with the broccoli. But it doesn't work that way.

Vitamin and mineral supplements weren't created to take the place of nutritious foods. For one thing, scientists still don't know whether the nutrients in supplements act the same way as the nutrients in food. And researchers are finding more and more evidence that foods contain essential substances that don't come in any capsule.

Boring and old-fashioned as it may sound, the best way to get the nutrients you need is by eating a well-balanced diet. According to the American Medical Association, if you're a healthy adult man or woman who's not pregnant or breastfeeding, and you're eating a well-balanced diet, you don't require supplements at all.

From time to time, hectic schedules, travel, or illness may wreak havoc with your diet. That's when supplements can come in handy. Some people also take supplements as a sort of insurance policy—*in addition to, rather than instead of, a good diet.* Women, in particular, have trouble getting enough bone-saving calcium in their diet, so they may be well advised to take a daily calcium supplement—if that's what the doctor orders.

motes healthy skin, helps eliminate toxins, regulates mood.

**What it may do:** protect the heart by reducing overall blood cholesterol levels and increasing the proportion of HDL ("good") cholesterol. It may also help prevent cancer, though scientists don't yet know how; however, studies have shown a relationship between niacin deficiency and cell malignancy.

**RDA:** 20 milligrams.

**Where to find it:** legumes, nuts, milk, cheese, eggs, green leafy vegetables, artichokes, asparagus, peas, potatoes, enriched cereals, liver, meat, swordfish, and chicken.

## Vitamin $B_6$—Pyridoxine

**What it does:** helps make protein, release stored glucose, and produce niacin, all of which are essential to growth, energy production, and red blood cell production.

**What it may do:** protect against heart disease by breaking down the amino acid homocysteine. Studies show that people with the highest levels of homocysteine in their blood are three times more likely to develop heart disease than those with low levels. $B_6$ may also boost the immune system, particularly among elderly people; researchers found that elderly people with low $B_6$ levels had less active immune systems.

**RDA:** 1.6 milligrams for women; 2 milligrams for men.

**Where to find it:** turkey, seafood, walnuts and other nuts, sesame seeds, wheat germ, legumes, leafy green vegetables, avocado, watercress, Brussels sprouts, cauliflower, cabbage, bananas, cantaloupe, enriched cereals, molasses, and milk.

## Vitamin $B_{12}$—Cobalamin

**What it does:** converts food into energy, helps produce red blood cells, aids in manufacture of genetic material (DNA and RNA), protects nerves, and helps the body utilize folic acid.

**What it may do:** protect against lung cancer caused by smoking; studies have shown that $B_{12}$ and folic acid may help reduce the number of precancerous cells in the body. Vitamin $B_{12}$ may also improve neurological function in the elderly, improving mood, memory, and balance.

**RDA:** 6.0 micrograms.

**Where to find it:** in all animal foods, especially liver, as well as seafood, milk, yogurt, eggs, mushrooms, tempeh, and enriched cereals.

## Vitamin $B_7$—Biotin

**What it does:** metabolizes protein and fat.
**What it may do:** prevent hair loss; strengthen nails.
**RDA:** 0.3 milligrams.
**Where to find it:** eggs, liver, wheat germ, nuts, oats, snow peas, artichokes, and mushrooms; it's also manufactured in the body.

## Vitamin $B_9$—Folic Acid

**What it does:** converts food into energy; helps produce red blood cells; aids growth and development; maintains immune system; works with vitamin $B_{12}$ to make genetic material (DNA); and protects against the neural tube birth defects spina bifida and anencephaly.
**What it may do:** help prevent cervical cancer; researchers theorize that folic acid in red blood cells may protect against HPV-16, a virus linked to this type of cancer. It has also been linked to reduced risk of colon and rectal cancers.
**RDA:** 400 micrograms; pregnant women, and women considering pregnancy, must be especially careful to get at least the RDA.
**Where to find it:** legumes; peanuts and other nuts; whole grains; fortified breakfast cereals; leafy green vegetables—especially watercress, parsley, spinach, and endive; raw beets; liver; and seafood.

## Vitamin $B_5$—Pantothenic Acid

**What it does:** metabolizes protein, fat, and carbohydrates; promotes growth; pantothenate supplements lower blood cholesterol levels.

**What it may do:** help treat rheumatoid arthritis.
**RDA:** 10 milligrams.
**Where to find it:** in most foods (except sugar, fats, and alcohol); best sources include wheat germ, legumes, avocado, mushrooms, dried apricots, pears, dates, whole grains, eggs, and liver.

## Vitamin C

**What it does:** helps form and maintain connective tissue; promotes growth and bone and tooth formation; helps the body absorb iron; promotes healing; enhances disease resistance by acting as an antioxidant.
**What it may do:** protect against many forms of cancer, including cancer of the stomach, pancreas, cervix, bladder, lungs, breasts, mouth, and esophagus; as well as childhood brain tumors (which are linked to low levels of vitamin C in the mother); prevent cataracts by preventing cell oxidation; help prevent heart disease by minimizing plaque buildup in the arteries, increasing levels of other antioxidants, and increasing levels of HDL ("good") cholesterol. High levels of C are also associated with lower blood pressure, thus reducing the risk of heart attack and stroke.
**RDA:** 60 milligrams.
**Where to find it:** citrus fruit, guava, black currants, strawberries, tomatoes, potatoes, cauliflower, peppers, and leafy green vegetables (especially when eaten raw).

## Vitamin D

**What it does:** promotes growth and aids in bone, tooth, and nail formation by helping the body absorb calcium.
**What it may do:** help prevent osteoporosis when

taken in combination with calcium. Vitamin D may also help prevent colon cancer, though it is not yet clear why; researchers have found, however, that colon cancer rates are higher in cold climates, where there is less sunlight.

**RDA:** 400 IUs. ***Warning:*** more than 25 micrograms, or 1,000 IUs, of vitamin D per day can be toxic.

**Where to find it:** the body manufactures most vitamin D when the skin is exposed to sunlight; it's also found in fortified milk and milk products, fatty fish such as salmon and sardines, and eggs (in small quantities).

## Vitamin E

**What it does:** protects nerves and cell membranes; maintains joint and ligament health; improves immunity; acts as an antioxidant, shielding cells from damage.

**What it may do:** guard against cancer by protecting cells and enhancing the immune system. Vitamin E is also strongly linked to lowering the risk for heart disease and stroke by preventing blood clots and preventing damage from oxidants, which help form plaque in the arteries; studies have found that high doses of vitamin E improve the outcome of open-heart surgery. It has been found to reduce arthritis pain and improve mobility, and may also slow the effects of aging.

**RDA:** 30 IUs.

**Where to find it:** nuts and seeds, especially sunflower seeds, pine nuts, hazelnuts, almonds, and peanuts; wheat germ, avocado, broccoli, asparagus, sweet potatoes, vegetable oil, whole-grain cereals, oats, and brown rice.

## RDAs and Megadoses

If you decide to take a vitamin/mineral supplement, the Food and Nutrition Board of the National Research Council recommends avoiding supplements that exceed 100 percent of the Recommended Daily Allowance. High doses of vitamins A, D, and E, and many minerals, can seriously harm your vital organs, and can also interfere with the absorption of other nutrients.

Almost all major health organizations agree, however, that the current RDAs are too low. The RDAs reflect the amount of each nutrient that's required to *avoid deficiency;* they do not indicate the amount of each nutrient that will promote optimal health. Researchers are currently working to establish new numbers for the essential nutrients based on recent findings that higher levels may offer myriad benefits.

Vitamin and mineral dosage is a complicated and controversial issue. Many "alternative medicine" practitioners, as well as some mainstream health experts, believe that so-called megadoses of certain vitamins, such as C, can do no harm—and may do wonders to fight cancer, AIDS, and other diseases. For now, however, unless your health practitioner recommends high doses of nutrients to fight a disease or other illness, you are well advised to wait for conclusive evidence about the benefits and perils of megadoses.

## Vitamin K

**What it does:** forms proteins that aid in blood clotting and other essential bodily functions. At least half the daily requirement is manufactured in the body.
**What it may do:** help prevent osteoporosis by aiding calcium retention.
**RDA:** 65 to 80 micrograms.
**Where to find it:** dairy products; vegetables, particularly green cabbage, Brussels sprouts, spinach, cauliflower, peas, and carrots; liver; and beans.

# Vital Minerals

Like vitamins, minerals are vital to keeping energy flowing through our bodies. They are found in enzymes and hormones, and are used to break down carbohydrates and fats. There are over three dozen known minerals, but only nineteen are known to be essential for our health. Most of these are needed only in trace amounts, but they're needed nonetheless. Below are some of the most common minerals, why you need them, and the best places to find them.

## Calcium

**What it does:** forms and maintains strong bones and teeth; maintains heart and other muscle function; aids in blood clotting; maintains cell membranes; helps conduct nerve impulses to and from the brain.

**What it may do**: retard osteoporosis (bone loss). Some studies show that insufficient calcium intake in adolescence can lead to bone loss in later life; others indicate that older women can stave off osteoporosis by consuming a high-calcium diet. Calcium may also lower blood pressure and cholesterol levels, helping prevent heart attack and stroke. Preliminary research indicates it may also help prevent colon and other cancers. Milk and other calcium-rich foods are an old folk remedy for PMS; preliminary studies indicate that a high-calcium diet may reduce PMS symptoms such as headache, irritability, and depression.

**RDA:** for adults up to age twenty-five, 1,200 milligrams; for adults over twenty-five, 800 milligrams.

**Where to find it:** milk, yogurt, tofu, canned salmon and sardines (with bones), leafy green

## Calcium Alert

Getting enough calcium is essential, both for maintaining a healthy body now and for reducing the future risk of osteoporosis; older women are particularly vulnerable to this brittle-bone disease, which can make your bones break as easily as twigs.

Although calcium is found in a wide variety of foods, it can be tricky to get enough because your body can't utilize it unless it has enough of other nutrients, such as phosphorus and magnesium, and hormones, such as estrogen. And any of the following can interfere with its absorption:

- consuming caffeine (more than two cups of coffee a day), soda, or alcohol (more than two glasses of wine or one mixed drink a day)
- smoking
- eating large amounts of protein
- eating lots of salty foods

The RDA for people over twenty-five is 800 milligrams, but the National Institutes of Health advocates an optimal intake of 1,000 milligrams for both men and women, and 1,500 for women who are pregnant or postmenopausal (and not on hormone replacement therapy).

The best bet is to eat a diet high in calcium-rich foods and take a calcium supplement to be sure you're getting all you need. There are many low-fat, high-nutrition choices:

- vegetables such as kale and broccoli
- low-fat yogurt and skim milk
- mineral water, which contains calcium

Another important factor is exercise: weight-bearing exercise such as walking, running, biking, and weight-training help keep your bones strong. And be sure to get out in the sunlight whenever you can—exposure to the sun makes your body produce vitamin D, which helps you absorb calcium.

vegetables, fortified breakfast cereals, almonds, and whole-wheat bread. Calcium is best absorbed when taken along with magnesium.

## Chromium

**What it does:** works with insulin to metabolize sugar, helping to maintain stable glucose levels.
**What it may do:** help prevent heart disease and stroke by raising levels of HDL cholesterol.
**RDA:** none established; experts estimate 50 to 200 micrograms.
**Where to find it:** meat, seafood, legumes, whole-grain cereal, nuts, brewer's yeast, and grape juice.

## Copper

**What it does:** maintains enzyme and immune systems; helps keep bones, nerves, and blood vessels healthy; plays an essential role in red blood cell formation.
**What it may do:** help treat arthritis—recent studies show that the old folk remedy for arthritis, copper bracelets, actually may help relieve stiffness and pain. Researchers have also found that copper in combination with anti-inflammatory drugs reduces arthritis symptoms. Copper may also help dissolve blood clots, which are considered a cause of heart disease.
**RDA:** 2 milligrams.
**Where to find it:** red meat, liver, oysters and other shellfish, wheat germ, whole-grain cereals, nuts and seeds, prunes, and olive oil.

## Iodine

**What it does:** maintains function of thyroid gland and thyroid hormones, which regulate more than one hundred enzyme systems involved in essential

functions such as metabolic rate, growth, and reproduction.
**RDA:** 150 micrograms.
**Where to find it:** saltwater fish, shellfish, seaweed, kelp, and iodized salt.

## Iron

**What it does:** transports oxygen to the cells, produces hemoglobin and red blood cell corpuscles. Too little iron in the system can cause anemia, fatigue, and depression.
**RDA:** 18 milligrams; too much iron can be toxic and increases the risk of heart disease.
**Where to find it:** red meat, liver, pork, poultry, oily fish (especially sardines), shellfish, tofu, legumes, leafy green vegetables, dried apricots, prunes, and molasses.

## Magnesium

**What it does:** maintains bones; helps produce energy from food; metabolizes vitamins and other minerals; helps regulate body temperature; prevents buildup of calcium and sodium, which can restrict blood flow; and as magnesium oxide (milk of magnesia), works as a laxative.
**What it may do:** because it regulates calcium and sodium, which can interfere with blood flow, magnesium may help protect against high blood pressure and thus reduce the risk of heart attack and stroke; a recent study showed a link between non-insulin-dependent diabetes, and low magnesium levels; another study found that magnesium supplements lowered blood pressure in people with this form of diabetes.
**RDA:** 250 to 350 milligrams; for pregnant and lactating women, 300 to 355 milligrams.

**Where to find it:** prunes, apricots, bananas, leafy green vegetables, meat, shrimp, soybeans, milk, whole-grain cereals, wheat germ, nuts and seeds.

## Manganese

**What it does:** builds bones; helps produce energy from food; helps produce fatty acids and cholesterol; maintains the nervous system; aids in the production of sex hormones; acts as an antioxidant.
**What it may do:** help prevent cancer and heart disease through its antioxidant function.
**RDA:** none established; experts recommend 2.5 to 5 milligrams.
**Where to find it:** tea, whole-grain cereals, eggs, nuts (especially pine nuts, macadamias, hazelnuts, and walnuts), peas, beets, leafy green vegetables, tofu and other soy products.

## Phosphorus

**What it does:** maintains muscle and nerve function; builds strong bones and teeth, helps produce energy from food; and helps form genetic material, cell membranes, and enzymes.
**RDA:** 1 gram.
**Where to find it:** almost all foods—calcium-rich foods are the best source.

## Potassium

**What it does:** balances body fluids, maintains nervous system.
**What it may do:** reduce high blood pressure—research has shown that patients given higher levels of dietary potassium were able to reduce their use of blood pressure medication by more than 50 percent.
**RDA:** 3,500 milligrams.

**Where to find it:** white and sweet potatoes, bananas, dried apricots and prunes, orange juice, lima beans and other legumes, milk, and plain yogurt.

## Selenium

**What it does:** protects cells from attack; helps control cholesterol; helps to protect the body by detoxifying potential carcinogens.
**What it may do:** protect against cancer—studies show that states with the highest levels of selenium in their soil (and thus in their local produce) have the lowest cancer rates. Selenium may also protect the heart—similar studies show that states with the lowest levels of selenium in their soil have the highest rates of stroke. Extra selenium may also improve male fertility, since low levels of the mineral reduce it.
**RDA:** 50 to 100 micrograms; cancer experts recommend at least 200 micrograms a day to protect against carcinogens.
**Where to find it:** red meat, chicken, eggs, shellfish and other seafood, whole grains, nuts (especially Brazil nuts), and broccoli.

## Sodium

**What it does:** helps maintain a normal balance of body fluids; maintains muscle and nerve function.
**RDA:** 2,400 milligrams.
**Where to find it:** almost all foods.

## Zinc

**What it does:** aids in growth, tissue formation, and healing; maintains the immune system; aids the action of various enzymes; helps the male reproductive system mature; and helps regulate appetite.
**What it may do:** because it is heavily concentrated in the prostate gland, zinc is linked to production

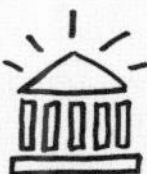

**SMART SOURCES**

These titles offer more useful information on micronutrients:

*Heinerman's Encyclopedia of Nature's Vitamins and Minerals*
by John Heinerman

*Getting the Most Out of Your Vitamins and Minerals*
by Jack Challem

*The Complete Book of Vitamin and Mineral Counts*
by Corinne T. Netzer

## Sodium Smarts

There's lots of confusion about sodium and salt. On the one hand, sodium is one of the minerals essential to your body's health. On the other hand, salt (sodium chloride) is bad for you—or is it?

Sodium is the main component of the body's extracellular fluids and helps carry nutrients into the cells; it also helps regulate other body functions, such as blood pressure and fluid volume. However, your body needs only a very small amount.

For a while there was widespread panic about salt—the dietary form of sodium—and the salt shaker was banished from many a table. But these days, many scientists agree that salt's been unfairly maligned. If you don't have high blood pressure, and are not at risk for it, you needn't worry about sprinkling a bit of salt on your food. But if you *are* at risk, you need to keep your salt intake at a strict minimum; hypertension can lead to heart attacks, kidney disease, and strokes. Some health experts also warn that excess salt intake makes your kidneys work too hard to get rid of the excess, and results in a loss of calcium.

One teaspoon of salt provides about 2,300 milligrams of sodium, so it's easy to consume more than the RDA of 2,400 milligrams, or even the more generous 4,000 milligrams recommended by other experts. Some 75 percent of the sodium Americans consume comes from processed foods—bread, cheese, canned foods, and more. So pushing away the salt shaker at home or at a restaurant won't help much.

To reduce your salt intake, try the following:

- Check for hidden sources of salt in your diet by reading nutrition labels when you shop.
- Stick to unprocessed foods as much as possible; they're better for your health.
- If you need to add salt when cooking, do it at the end; you're likely to add much less.
- Try substituting herbs and spices; they're a healthier alternative for flavor.
- Cut down gradually; you may find yourself losing your taste for salt.

When you do eat salty foods, increase your potassium intake by eating lots of fresh fruits and vegetables—potassium may help reduce blood pressure.

of semen and to testosterone metabolism; therefore, researchers believe higher intake of zinc may be effective against male infertility as well as enlargement of the prostate gland, which can lead to prostate cancer. Zinc supplements may also help reduce the duration of the common cold, though evidence is not conclusive.
**RDA:** 15 milligrams.
**Where to find it:** meat, poultry, oysters and other shellfish, eggs, hard cheeses, whole-wheat bread, legumes, garlic, ginger, wheatgerm, almonds, pumpkin seeds, and sunflower seeds.

***F.Y.I.***

Americans' average daily fiber intake is about half that recommended by the American Heart Association and other major organizations.

# Two Other Essentials: Fiber and Water

Fiber and water are overlooked components of the nutritional nexus. Not enough people concern themselves with getting sufficient quantities of either, or both, or even know what constitutes a sufficient quantity. But shortchanging fiber and water in your diet is like forgetting to change the oil in your car—it'll screw up the whole works.

## Fiber Matters

Fiber contains no calories or nutrients, and it passes through your body in undigested form. So what's the point of eating it? Well, for one thing, fiber is an excellent aid to digestion (as long as you consume it in moderation—more on that later). And it also helps prevent constipation. In fact, many people think about fiber only in this

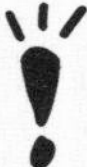

**SMART MOVE**

Truly a man ahead of his time, Sylvester Graham, the man who gave the world graham crackers, was already extolling the virtues of fiber back in the nineteenth century. Graham was convinced that fiber was the most healthful component of grains, fruits, and beans—a theory that raised more than a few eyebrows. Today researchers are finding more and more evidence that Graham was on the right track: fiber ranks right up there with vitamins and minerals as a health and healing essential.

context, and reach for Metamucil or another high-fiber packaged product when they're suffering "irregularity." But that's a mistake you shouldn't make, because fiber does many more good things for your health.

There are two types of fiber:

**Soluble fiber,** found in foods such as oat bran, broccoli, and apples, slows the movement of food through the intestine.

**Insoluble fiber,** found in foods such as wheat bran, dried beans such as kidney and pinto, and celery, speeds up the movement of food through the intestine.

Although the two functions seem to cancel each other out, you need both soluble and insoluble fiber to keep you healthy. You don't need to worry about which kind you're eating; if you eat a wide array of fruits, vegetables, and whole grains, you'll get plenty of both.

Getting plenty is your goal: in addition to performing important digestive functions, fiber is known to prevent certain health problems and diseases. For example, fiber is known to do, or is strongly suspected of doing, the following:

- Help prevent hemorrhoids. Hemorrhoids are very uncommon in countries where people eat high-fiber diets.
- Lower blood cholesterol levels.
- Lower the risk of heart disease.
- Help prevent colon cancer.
- Help diabetics control their blood sugar levels; high-fiber foods take longer to break down into sugars.

For all these reasons, the National Cancer Institute and the American Dietetic Association recommend that Americans consume lots of it: 20 to 35 grams of fiber a day. Somewhere in the middle of that range is a good place to start; too much can lead to bloating and diarrhea. And remember, the more fiber you eat, the more water you should drink, to keep all that roughage moving through your body.

The best sources of fiber are the same foods that are healthiest for you overall:

- fresh and dried fruits
- raw vegetables
- legumes
- whole-grain and rye breads
- buckwheat, bulgur, barley, and other whole grains
- oatmeal
- wheat and oat bran—just two tablespoons provide close to the minimum daily requirement for fiber

**F.Y.I.**

A good way to tell if you're drinking enough water and other fluids is to check the color of your urine. If it's medium to dark yellow, you need to drink more.

## Water Works

Water—be it bottled or plain old filtered tap water—is as vital to your health as oxygen. Water keeps your body hydrated, aids digestion and metabolism, and helps flush out waste and toxins. Without enough water the body becomes dehydrated, leading to: kidney problems, cystitis (a painful, stinging infection of the bladder or urethra), skin problems, migraines and other headaches. Yet many people still drink much less water than they should.

### How Much Do You Need?

Your body's water supply must be constantly replenished because you lose at least ten cups a day through breathing, perspiration, evaporation,

## Water Wisdom

These days, choosing water is nearly as complicated as choosing wine. Here's the lowdown on the healthiest options:

**Mineral water** comes from a single underground source, is required by law to be free of harmful bacteria and chemicals, and must maintain a consistent mineral content. It can be filtered and exposed to ultraviolet light, but it cannot be disinfected or sterilized in any other way. It can be sparkling or still.

Mineral water is your best bet because it's carefully monitored for purity; it's consistently good-tasting; and it contains health-enhancing nutrients including calcium and magnesium, albeit in tiny amounts. But be aware that it also contains sodium; some brands have more than others. If you have high blood pressure or heart disease, check the label.

**Spring** and **table water** may come from a spring or from a tap connected to your area's water system—bottlers are not required to identify the source, and they often mix water from different sources. These waters need to meet the standards set for tap water; beyond that, there are no requirements, so bottlers can do what they want. Beware, too, of **restaurant bottled water,** which is often just filtered tap water sold at outrageous prices.

Filtered **tap water,** therefore, may be just as good a bet, and it's certainly cheaper. Filtering the water will eliminate any unpleasant chlorine taste; another option is boiling, then chilling your water. Still, the fact that nearly all tap water is recycled (over and over) and is often contaminated by chemicals that seep into the ground makes many people opt for bottled water. Remember, buy mineral water, or you may be paying a premium for the same stuff.

and excretion. By the time you experience thirst, your body is already dehydrated. So don't wait until you feel thirsty to drink water; rather, make water intake a habit.

You should strive to drink a minimum of 64 ounces of water (8 cups) a day. You can also replenish a certain amount of water by drinking other liquids, such as fruit juices, and eating fruits and vegetables—cucumbers, watermelons, and other juicy choices.

# Phytonutrients: The New Frontier

Phytonutrients, also known as phytochemicals or functional foods, are chemicals or nutrients found in plant foods. If you've never heard of them, you're not alone. Unlike vitamins and minerals, which have long been touted for their health-giving properties, phytonutrients are just coming into the nutritional spotlight, and researchers are just beginning to discover their powerful health benefits.

Phytonutrients' most basic function is protecting the health of plants, not people. Some guard against plant viruses, bacteria, and other threats. Others repel bugs and other predators. Yet research shows that these same nutrients are effective against human threats as well: when you eat plant foods, you get phytonutrient-powered protection against a whole range of health woes—and researchers are adding to the list each day.

Based on what's known so far, phytonutrients appear to serve three major functions in the human body: they act as antioxidants; they regulate hormone levels; and they eliminate toxins.

## Antioxidant Action

Most phytonutrients help fight disease by acting as antioxidants. They protect the body from free radicals—oxygen molecules that have lost an electron due to damage from sunlight, pollution, or other natural or environmental causes. These damaged molecules attempt to latch on to other, healthy molecules in order to scavenge their electrons; when they succeed, the healthy molecules become damaged and turn into free radicals as well. If this

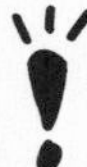

**SMART MOVE**

"We now see a renewed awareness and interest in returning to nature to address the two leading causes of death that plague our society: cancer and cardiovascular disease," says Leslie Jacobs, an internist in Las Vegas, Nevada. "It has not, of course, reached a point that we would give up our pharmaceutical arsenal and write prescriptions to our patient's grocer, nor would we have our patients take a clove of garlic, two chili peppers, and call us in the morning. However, we do sense a willingness among many professionals in the medical community to address health issues from a preventive stance through proper diet, nutritional supplementation, exercise, and elimination of bad habits."

process continues, the accumulation of damaged molecules wreaks havoc on your body, leading to permanent damage and disease. Free radical damage can cause everything from hardening of the arteries—setting the stage for heart disease—to cancer to premature aging.

Phytonutrients create a protective barrier between your body's cells and free radicals. They provide electrons to the free radicals, thus stabilizing them and preventing further damage.

## Hormone Regulation

Phytonutrients also help maintain healthful levels of various hormones, which in turn help keep disease at bay.

One example, and one that has garnered a great deal of attention, is phytonutrients' effect on estrogen levels. Evidence has shown that women are at higher risk of breast cancer when they have high estrogen levels. Researchers believe that a diet high in certain phytonutrients called isoflavones may help reduce breast cancer risk; these substances, which are very similar to natural estrogen, appear to supplant excess estrogen in the body, thus restoring estrogen levels to the safe zone.

## Toxin Elimination

Another way in which phytonutrients protect is by helping to detoxify carcinogens—cancer-causing chemicals—and flush them out of the body. The phytonutrients attack "bad" enzymes that help activate toxins, while increasing production of "good" enzymes that find and detoxify the carcinogens.

## Where to Find Them

Phytonutrients are not available in any pill or potion—though researchers hope they will be someday soon, so people can receive their benefits in concentrated form. Until then, there's only one way to get them: through fruits, vegetables, and grains.

# The Emerging Superstars

Hundreds of phytonutrients have been identified so far; but as yet, little or nothing is known about many of them. But those that have been studied show tremendous promise as health and healing dynamos. Below are some of the major finds.

### Allylic Sulfides

**Best sources:** onions and garlic; also found in lower concentrations in leeks, shallots, and chives. Released when plants are cut or bruised.
**What they do:** fight bacterial, viral, and fungal infections; aid circulation; detoxify the liver; may help prevent heart disease by lowering cholesterol and fat levels; lower blood sugar levels; may protect against cancer, particularly stomach cancer, by detoxifying cancer-causing chemicals.

### Phenols

**Best sources:** almost all fruits, vegetables, and grains, as well as green and black teas.

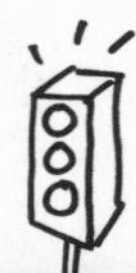

**WHAT MATTERS, WHAT DOESN'T**

### What Matters

- Eating a variety of foods to obtain the full range of nutrients.
- Taking a vitamin/mineral supplement when you can't eat right.
- Avoiding too much of any nutrient; some can be toxic in high doses.

### What Doesn't

- Getting every nutrient every day; it's what you eat over a period of days and weeks that matters.
- Treating the RDAs as gospel; many researchers think the numbers are too low.

**What they do:** act as antioxidants; prevent blood clots; prevent inflammation; activate enzymes that fight cancer.

## Flavonoids

**Best sources:** onions, kale, endive, broccoli, citrus fruits, cranberries, apples (with peels), grape juice, and red wine.
**What they do:** act as antioxidants, fighting allergies, inflammation, free radicals, toxins, microbes, ulcers, viruses, and tumors; prevent blood clotting and protect against heart disease; protect veins; lower levels of harmful estrogen, reducing the risk of estrogen-induced breast cancer; may help prevent cataracts. A subgroup of flavonoids, called anthocyanidins, strengthen collagen (used to make skin and other tissues, tendons, and ligaments) and scavenge free radicals in tissue fluids—this particularly benefits athletes because heavy exercise generates free radicals.

## Isoflavones

**Best sources:** chickpeas, lentils, kidney beans, soybeans and soy products.
**What they do:** block tumor-causing enzymes; lower levels of harmful estrogen; may help reduce risk of breast, prostate, and uterine cancers.

## Carotenoids

**Best sources:** yellow, orange, and red fruits and vegetables, including: cantaloupe, pink grapefruit, tomatoes, and carrots; also broccoli, spinach, and other greens.
**What they do:** act as antioxidants; may help prevent prostate, colorectal, lung, breast, and uterine

cancers; may prevent arteriosclerosis, heart disease, and stroke

## Indoles

**Best sources:** cauliflower, broccoli, cabbage, and mustard greens.
**What they do:** lower levels of harmful estrogen, reducing the risk of estrogen-induced breast cancer; activate enzymes that detoxify carcinogens, particularly in the gastrointestinal tract.

## Phytosterols

**Best sources:** found in most plants, particularly green and yellow vegetables.
**What they do:** block absorption of dietary cholesterol and help excrete it from the body; block the development of tumors in the breast, colon, and prostate; reduce inflammation.

## Saponins

**Best sources:** tomatoes, potatoes, chickpeas, soybeans, spinach, asparagus, nuts, and oats.
**What they do:** stimulate the immune system; block absorption of dietary cholesterol and help excrete it from the body; may help prevent heart disease and some cancers.

## Glucosinolates

**Best sources:** cauliflower, broccoli, cabbage, and other cruciferous vegetables.
**What they do:** activate enzymes that detoxify the liver; block enzymes that promote tumor growth, particularly in the stomach, esophagus, lungs, colon, and breasts; regulate white blood cells, which protect the immune system.

**F.Y.I.**

Tomatoes contain an estimated ten thousand phytonutrients.

# The Key Is Balance

If you eat a well-balanced diet, you're guaranteed to get the full complement—and the full benefit—of macronutrients and micronutrients. But some foods offer more potent nutrient packages than others; in the following chapter you'll learn about the very best choices for everyday eating.

**THE BOTTOM LINE**

All the components of food—fat, carbohydrates, and protein; vitamins, minerals, fiber, and phytonutrients—work as a team to keep your body in peak condition. If you choose to take vitamin and mineral supplements, be sure you do use them as *supplements* to a good diet, not as replacements. Pills can't possibly provide all the nutrients you get from food; there are no shortcuts to good nutrition and optimum health.

CHAPTER 3

# The Super Foods

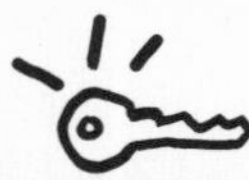

**THE KEYS**

- Eat an abundance of the top twenty-nine foods for peak health.
- Each food is packed with essential vitamins, minerals, and other nutrients in each food.
- Learn which foods can help you fight disease and other ailments.
- Buying, storing, and preparing foods correctly will guarantee optimum nutrition.
- Incorporate healing foods into your everyday menus with easy, delicious recipes.

Winnowing down the bounty of healing foods is no easy task; all fruits, vegetables, and grains, as well as many animal products, have their own healthy array of nutrients and benefits. And eating the greatest possible array of nutritious foods is the best way to ensure optimal health.

That said, the choices below represent the best of the best: foods that provide the most nutritional bang per bite, without dangerous fat or excess calories. But they are more than health superstars; all these foods are so delicious that you will want to give them a regular slot on your menus. And when it comes to feeling your best, taste matters every bit as much as nutrition: fresh, great-tasting food is a boon to both body and soul.

**Note:** Garlic and ginger, two top healing foods, are found in chapter 5, "Healing Herbs and Spices."

## Almonds

- Lower cholesterol levels.
- May help lower risk of heart disease.

Don't make the common mistake of avoiding nuts because they're too rich in fat and calories. That would be a particular shame where almonds are concerned; they're one of the most concentrated, easy-to-eat sources of energy and nutrients.

### Good Fat Fights Bad Cholesterol

It's true that almonds, like other nuts, are no prize when it comes to calories and fat content. They contain 13 grams of fat per ounce. However, that fat is

87 percent monounsaturated fat, the kind that helps lower cholesterol and thus may protect you against heart disease. Studies have shown that people who add 3 ounces of almonds to their daily diet have an average 10 percent drop in cholesterol.

Almonds offer other heart-protecting substances as well. Almonds are high in vitamin E, which helps keep artery-clogging plaque at bay, thereby reducing your risk of high blood pressure, heart attacks, and stroke. If you eat just an ounce of almonds a day, you'll double the average vitamin E intake.

**F.Y.I.**

Many researchers believe that vitamin E protects the heart only when consumed at levels well above the RDA.

## Beneficial Minerals

That's not the end of the good heart news. Two minerals found in almonds, copper and magnesium, appear to help regulate cholesterol. And magnesium may also help lower blood pressure and regulate heart rhythms.

Almonds are also an excellent source of calcium; they contain more of this mineral than any other nut, and are in fact one of the richest nonanimal sources of it. In addition to its well-known bone-strengthening benefits, calcium helps regulate heartbeat and normalize blood pressure.

## More Good News

A few almonds also provide a hefty shot of protein and other nutrients. Almonds are 20 percent protein—ounce for ounce, they offer a third more protein than eggs. An ounce of almonds contains about 6 grams of protein and the same amount of fiber; because fiber slows down the body's use of energy, almonds are a great source of slow-burning fuel (which explains why they're rarely absent from trail mix).

Finally, as if that's not enough: Almond oil is a wonderful skin soother.

**F.Y.I.**

Almonds contain two kinds of acid—oxalic and phytic acids—which make it difficult to retain minerals in your body. Eating a food rich in vitamin C along with almonds will help you absorb the maximum nutrients.

**Tips:**
Choose unblanched rather than blanched (skinless) almonds; they are higher in nutrients. Store almonds in the refrigerator if you plan to use them within a few weeks; for long-term storage, use the freezer.

## Apples

- Lower blood cholesterol levels
- Treat constipation and diarrhea
- Help control diabetes
- Strengthen immune system
- May lower risk of heart disease
- May help prevent cancer

We all know apples are supposed to be good for your health, yet it was only recently that researchers discovered their benefits.

### The Pectin Connection

The answer lies in apples' storehouse of fiber and potent phytonutrients.

One medium unpeeled apple provides 3.5 grams of fiber, more than 10 percent of the daily fiber intake recommended by experts (without the peel it provides 2.7 grams). The insoluble fiber in apples works like bran fiber, attaching to cholesterol in the digestive tract and helping to sweep it out of the body, thus reducing the risk of clogged arteries, heart attack, and stroke.

But that's not all. Apples also contain a form of soluble fiber called pectin, which may help reduce the amount of natural cholesterol produced in the liver. Not only does pectin target cholesterol; it also specifically zooms in on LDL cholesterol, the kind that clogs arteries and keeps blood from reaching vital organs.

How much good can apples do your cholesterol level—and your heart? Researchers have found that eating two apples a day can lower cholesterol levels by up to 16 percent. Another much-cited study showed that men who consumed an apple a day, along with two tablespoons of onion and four cups of tea, had a 32 percent lower risk of heart attack than those who ate fewer apples.

## Cancer Protection

Apple skin contains a large supply of a compound called quercetin, an antioxidant that may help prevent heart disease.

The antioxidants quercetin and vitamin C help prevent the free radical damage that can lead to cancer.

Apples also get some of their cancer-fighting power from pectin. Researchers believe that pectin may attach itself to environmental pollutants that make their way into the body—substances such as lead and mercury—and help flush them out. And the insoluble fiber in apples may help prevent diverticulosis and colon cancer. By relieving constipation (see below), fiber also helps flush out dangerous substances in stools that might otherwise lead to cancer.

## Digestive Aid

The insoluble fiber in apples (a.k.a. roughage) helps relieve constipation, and as mentioned above, it thereby helps prevent colon cancer. At the same time, apples' *soluble* fiber helps treat diarrhea. (Some doctors prescribe the BRAT diet—bananas, rice,

**F.Y.I.**

The sugar in apples is mostly fructose, a simple sugar that's broken down slowly and helps keep blood sugar levels stable—so apples are good for diabetics, too.

The antioxidant vitamin C in apples helps strengthen the body's immune defenses.

Their fiber content helps fill you up, making them a great choice if you're trying to shed a few pounds.

The smell of apples has a calming effect on many people and even helps lower blood pressure.

apples, and toast—as a diarrhea remedy. Natural health practitioners also recommend grating an apple, letting it turn brown, and mixing it with a little honey as a remedy for diarrhea.)

Traditionally, apples have been used to treat upset stomach. And with good reason: apples contain malic and tartaric acids, which help digestion.

**Tips:**
Apples are most nutritious when eaten raw, though lightly cooked apples retain most of their nutrients. They are often treated with insecticides and coated with wax; scrub them before eating. But don't peel them; you'll lose a lot of their beneficial pectin and nutrients. If you're really worried about chemicals, buy organic apples.

# Apricots

- Lower cholesterol
- Help regulate blood pressure
- Protect eyesight
- May help fight cancer
- May lower risk of heart disease and stroke

Whether fresh or dried, apricots taste like a burst of pure sunshine. They also provide a burst of pure nutrition.

## Carotene Bonanza

Apricots are one of the top fruits for beta-carotene, as you can tell from a glance at their bright-orange color. Beta-carotene is just the beginning of the story; researchers have identified some 600 other carotenoids as well, and apricots contain an assort-

## Apricots: Fresh or Dried?

Both fresh and dried apricots are full of nutrients, but dried apricots have the edge. A half cup provides 100 percent of the RDA for this beta-carotene, versus 50 percent in three fresh apricots. They are also richer in potassium and fiber, and they make a good remedy for constipation.

Dried apricots are also higher in calories than fresh—three small fresh apricots contain about 50 calories; a half cup of dried apricots contains about 165 calories. That makes them a great source of concentrated energy (you'll find them in many a backpacker's pack) but also a food to be careful of when you're trying to lose weight; it's easy to eat a lot more than a half cup's worth.

Another point to consider: most commercial dried apricots are preserved with sulfur dioxide, which can trigger asthma attacks. If you are susceptible, read labels carefully (the FDA requires manufacturers to list sulfur dioxide or sulfites on the package) and rinse apricots thoroughly, or buy untreated apricots at natural food stores. However, be aware that unsulfured dried apricots lose most of their beta-carotene.

Best advice: eat all the fresh apricots you can during their brief summer season; they're uniquely delicious. The rest of the year, go with the dried.

ment of the most powerfully protective types that are available.

Studies show that people who eat foods high in antioxidant carotenes have lower cancer rates. And beta-carotene has also been found to prevent formation of plaque deposits in arteries, which can lead to coronary artery disease.

In the body, beta-carotene converts to vitamin A. An especially helpful nutrient for eye health, vitamin A protects the eyes from tissue-damaging free radicals that can cause cataracts and other vision problems. A study of more than fifty thousand nurses showed that women who got the most vitamin A in their diets reduced their risk of getting cataracts by more than one third.

**F.Y.I.**

Apricots are a good source of potassium, which helps prevent high blood pressure and maintains normal heart function.

The boron in apricots may help prevent osteoporosis in older women; boron helps the body retain beneficial estrogen, which in turn aids calcium absorption.

Apricots also contain iron, which is essential for the formation of red blood cells. Iron deficiency, particularly common in women, can lead to fatigue and weaken resistance to infection.

### Added Antioxidant Protection

Apricots are also a rich source of the compound lycopene, one of the strongest known antioxidants. Like beta-carotene, lycopene helps keep LDL cholesterol from sticking to artery walls, preventing arteriosclerosis, high blood pressure, and heart attacks.

**Tips:**
To improve iron absorption, eat dried apricots with foods rich in vitamin C. If you opt for fresh apricots, eat them while they are still somewhat firm to get the most nutrients; after their peak, the nutrients begin to break down.

## Bananas

- Help lower blood pressure
- Boost energy levels
- Help improve mood
- Relieve constipation and diarrhea
- Relieve acid indigestion and may help prevent ulcers
- May lower risk of heart disease and stroke

Bananas are known as nature's perfect fast food, and with good reason. Delicious, nutritious, and a great source of long-lasting energy, they're a favorite with everyone from infants to iron-pumping athletes.

### Potassium Plus

Bananas are among the best sources of potassium, a mineral that's essential for normal blood pressure and heart function. Potassium helps regulate fluid levels in the body and helps get rid of excess sodium, which can cause blood pressure to rise and in turn lead to heart attack and stroke.

## Stomach Protection

For many decades, scientists recognized that bananas have an antacid effect on the stomach but had no clear idea why. Recent studies have found that substances in bananas help strengthen cells in the stomach lining, creating a stronger barrier against corrosive digestive acids. Bananas also appear to stimulate the production of protective mucus and help kill off harmful bacteria. Thanks to all this protective power, bananas may be an effective tool for preventing and treating not only simple acid indigestion but also ulcers.

## Digestive Regulation

Bananas are a good source of the soluble fiber pectin, which helps slow digestion and regulate blood sugar levels. That and their complex carbohydrates make them an excellent source of steady-burning energy. Pectin also helps absorb excess fluids in the digestive tract, helping to prevent diarrhea; meanwhile, bananas' starch helps ease constipation.

**Tips:**
If your bananas tend to get overripe before you have a chance to eat them, try refrigerating them as soon as they become ripe. The skin will turn dark, but the inside will remain at peak ripeness for several days.

**F.Y.I.**

One banana contains over a quarter of the RDA of vitamin $B_6$, a nutrient that's helpful in preventing the depression and irritability that can accompany PMS.

Because bananas are high in carbohydrates, eating one or two ripe bananas can help raise levels of mood-lifting serotonin in the brain.

**F.Y.I.**

Spices such as ginger and dill may help reduce the gassy effect of beans.

# Beans/Legumes

- Lower cholesterol
- Maintain stable blood sugar levels
- May help prevent cancer
- May help prevent heart disease

Vegetarians have long relied on legumes—dried beans and peas—as a nutritious source of nonanimal protein. Meat eater or not, you'd be wise to do the same; lentils, chickpeas, and other beans have everything to offer the health-conscious eater.

## Fibrous Wonders

Legumes could double as cholesterol-lowering pills; they're high in soluble fiber, which helps trap cholesterol and remove it from the body, in turn reducing your risk of heart disease. In a recent study, men who were given a diet containing 4 ounces of pinto and navy beans daily reduced their total cholesterol by an average of 19 percent, and their LDL cholesterol by 24 percent.

Foods with high fiber content also help keep blood sugar levels stable, which helps control diabetes. Soluble fiber helps lead insulin into individual cells and out of the bloodstream, where it can cause problems. Eating just one-half cup of beans a day has been shown to significantly improve blood sugar control.

All that fiber, along with plentiful complex carbohydrates, also make legumes a great choice for anyone who wants steady, slow-burning energy. (The best fiber choices include: black-eyed peas, kidney beans, chickpeas, lima beans, and black beans.) And beans give you a full feeling that makes you unlikely to overdo it on other, less healthy foods.

## Anticancer Compounds

Beans contain compounds—lignans, saponins, isoflavones, phytic acid, and protease inhibitors—that have been shown to help prevent cancer. Protease inhibitors, for example, can stop normal cells from becoming cancerous in the early stages of cancer. And isoflavones help deactivate potent estrogens that can lead to breast cancer.

## Healthy Protein

Like meat, beans are loaded with protein; unlike meat, they're not loaded with fat and calories.

Beans contain incomplete rather than complete protein. That means the protein is missing some of the ingredients to make it usable in your body. No problem—just do what vegetarians have been doing for centuries: combine beans with a starch such as rice that provides a complementary protein. But although beans and starches make a natural combination, you don't have to have them together in order to obtain complete protein; as long as you get two complementary proteins during the course of the day, you'll be fine.

**Tips:**
Don't fret if there's never time to soak and cook beans: canned beans are just as nutritious as dried beans and will do just as much to help lower cholesterol. But if you use the canned kind, be sure to rinse them well first; they're packed in sodium-laden liquid.

**F.Y.I.**

A half-cup of black beans contains 32 percent of the RDA for folate, which can lower heart disease risk and prevent birth defects.

Beans contain useful amounts of iron; in fact, they have nearly the iron content of white meat or fish. That's very good news for women, who tend to be low in this mineral.

They're also a good source of potassium, which helps maintain heart health.

**F.Y.I.**

With its high vitamin C content, cabbage improves resistance to infections.

Raw cabbage juice is a traditional ulcer remedy, and studies have validated its effectiveness. Researchers think a substance called gefarnate may be responsible; it stimulates cells to produce a layer of mucus that protects the stomach from acid.

A one-cup serving of bok choy contains as much calcium as one-half cup of milk, making it a good food for building and maintaining strong bones and teeth. And it's the richest leafy green source of boron, which also helps preserve bone density.

# Bok Choy and Other Cabbages

- Speed ulcer healing and improve digestive health
- Help prevent cataracts
- Cut risk of birth defects
- May reduce risk of cancer
- May lower risk of heart disease and stroke

Cabbage is a nutritional king. A member of the cancer-fighting cruciferous family, it's loaded with protective compounds and useful nutrients. If you only eat it as mayo-drenched coleslaw at the family picnic, you're missing out on a bonanza of healing benefits.

## The Best of the Best

While all cabbages are good for you, some are even better.

Frequently used in stir-fries and other Asian dishes, bok choy, or Chinese cabbage, is higher in nutrients than regular cabbage. One cup of chopped bok choy contains almost the entire RDA for the antioxidant beta-carotene; it's also high in vitamin C and potassium, all of which are crucial to maintaining normal blood pressure and heart health.

Savoy cabbage is another standout; it, too, is high in disease-fighting beta-carotene, as well as in vitamin C.

## Cancer Fighters

Like other cruciferous vegetables, cabbage contains indoles, phytonutrients that seem to deactivate powerful estrogens that stimulate the growth of tumors, particularly in the breast. Another compound in bok choy, called brassinin, has also been linked to preventing breast tumors.

Studies have shown that a third compound in cabbage, called sulforaphane, is effective against both breast and colon cancers. Sulforaphane appears to increase production of enzymes that prevent tumors. It's been shown to reduce occurrence of breast tumors in laboratory animals by more than 40 percent. Sulforaphane also stimulates production of an enzyme called glutathione, which works to remove toxins from the colon, and eliminate them from the body before they can damage cells.

Savoy cabbage is particularly potent against cancer because it contains indoles, sulforaphane, and at least four other phytonutrients that help eliminate toxins.

**Tips:**
Never boil bok choy or other cabbages—you'll lose half the nutrients (and all the flavor) that way. Eating it raw is best; try it in place of some of your regular salad greens, or make a low-fat coleslaw with vinaigrette.

**SMART DEFINITION**

**Cruciferous vegetables**

Also called crucifers, these vegetables are named for the cross shape of their four-petal flowers. Crucifers, which include broccoli, brussels sprouts, cabbage, cauliflower, kale, kohlrabi, mustard greens, rutabagas, and turnips, are strongly linked with lower rates of cancer.

# Broccoli

- Helps lowers risk of heart disease and stroke
- Lowers risk of birth defects
- Keeps digestive system running smoothly
- Maintains strong bones
- Helps prevent cataracts
- May reduce cancer risk

Broccoli is one of the most potent food "medicines" there is. If you've been shunning it since childhood,

**F.Y.I.**

With 36 grams of calcium per half cup (as well as zinc, which aids its absorption), broccoli is one of the best nonanimal sources of this bone-strengthening mineral. That makes it a particularly valuable choice for older women, who are prone to osteoporosis.

Broccoli is also a good source of fiber, which helps maintain digestion and prevent high cholesterol, colon and other cancers, and obesity.

It also supplies folate, a nutrient that helps prevent the birth defect spina bifida as well as cancer and heart disease; and potassium, which is essential for normal fluid balance, heart function, and blood pressure.

do your body a favor and try it again. Fresh, lightly steamed or stir-fried broccoli tastes nothing like the limp, overcooked stalks that once made you shudder. And while all cruciferous vegetables contain potent antidisease compounds, broccoli may be the best nutritional choice of the bunch.

## Cruciferous Compounds

Like other crucifers, broccoli contains compounds called indoles that help prevent tumor growth. Indoles help deactivate the potent estrogens that trigger tumors in cells, especially estrogen-sensitive breast cells. Another compound, sulforaphane, stimulates cells to produce some important carcinogen-fighting enzymes.

## Vital Antioxidants

Broccoli is bursting with antioxidants, which strengthen the immune system and help protect against cancer, heart disease, cataracts, and other illnesses. A half-cup serving of cooked broccoli provides nearly 100 percent of the RDA for vitamin C, as well as a good dose of beta-carotene and selenium. It also provides almost one-third of the RDA for vitamin E, which is crucial to heart health.

**Tips:**

Organic broccoli may be your best bet, since the dense broccoli florets can retain chemical residue even after rinsing. Raw broccoli is good, but cooked broccoli is even better. Lightly steaming or stir-frying it releases beneficial compounds.

If you can find broccoli sprouts in your supermarket, buy them! Studies have shown they contain twenty to fifty times the amount of protective nutrients found in mature broccoli.

# Carrots

- Lower blood cholesterol
- Improve night vision
- Help protect against food poisoning
- May help protect against cancer
- May help prevent heart disease and stroke

Your mother probably told you to eat your carrots to keep from going blind: a slight exaggeration, although carrots do help maintain night vision. But it's hard to exaggerate their other benefits.

## Carotene Kings

Carrots are a terrific source of the antioxidant beta-carotene; in fact, they are by far the best commonly consumed source of this essential nutrient. Just one raw carrot contains 13,500 IUs of beta-carotene, more than 250 percent of the RDA. High beta-carotene intake has been shown to decrease the rates of bladder, cervix, prostate, colon, larynx, and esophageal cancers by up to 50 percent, and to reduce the rate of postmenopausal breast cancer by 20 percent. Carrot consumption has also been shown to reduce the rate of lung cancer.

Until recently, scientists believed that beta-carotene alone was responsible for the fact that carrot eaters are far less likely to suffer from certain cancers; thus they figured that putting beta-carotene in a pill would produce the same effects. This proved not to be the case—much to the dismay of vitamin manufacturers.

Now scientists theorize that other substances in carrots may play a vital role as well. One prime contender is alpha-carotene, a lesser-known anti-

**F.Y.I.**

The average carrot contains 2.3 grams of fiber, much of it in the form of calcium pectate—a fiber that's particularly effective in reducing cholesterol. According to USDA researchers, two carrots a day may reduce total cholesterol levels by as much as 20 percent.

Thanks to their high antioxidant content, raw carrots can kill listeria and other food-poisoning organisms.

oxidant that carrots contain in abundance. A recent National Cancer Institute study found that lung cancer occurred more often in men with low intakes of alpha-carotene.

## Visionaries

Carrots earned their reputation as eyesight preservers thanks to their high vitamin A content. When beta-carotene converts to vitamin A in the body, it forms an eye pigment called rhodopsin that enables you to see in dim light. And beta-carotene's antioxidant effects also provide protection against cataracts and macular degeneration, the top cause of vision loss in older adults.

**Tips:**

Opt for whole carrots instead of carrot juice; that way you'll get the full fiber benefits.

If you buy carrots with the greenery intact, remove it before storing, or the green tops will suck out all the vitamins and moisture.

Peel all but organic carrots; carrots are especially likely to be treated with pesticides and other chemicals.

Beta-carotene is not destroyed by cooking; in fact, cooking releases more of the beneficial nutrient from fiber.

# Celery

- Helps reduce high blood pressure
- Acts as a diuretic, which may ease joint problems
- Soothes nerves
- May lower cancer risk

You may think of celery as the stalky equivalent of iceberg lettuce—something innocuous and low-calorie to crunch. In fact, unlike that pallid salad fare, celery, and celery seeds, are packed with healthy goodness—pretty remarkable in a food that's almost 90 percent water!

**F.Y.I.**

If you are sensitive to salt, don't go overboard eating celery. Too much might to more harm than good to your blood pressure, since celery contains 35 milligrams of sodium per stalk.

## Diuretic Action

Celery's diuretic properties have been known for centuries. By stimulating urine production, celery helps the body get rid of excess fluid and uric acid, which can aggravate joint pain associated with arthritis, rheumatism, and gout. Celery also contains insoluble fiber, which helps move other waste more quickly through and out of the body.

The combination of potassium and sodium in celery are essential to regulating fluid balance, which affects every part of the body.

## Cancer Prevention

Researchers have discovered a number of compounds in celery that act as antioxidants, helping to prevent cancer or cancer growth. Phenolic acids help stop free radicals from damaging normal cells and making them cancerous; they also help neutralize carcinogenic substances such as nitrosamines, which can be formed when you eat foods containing nitrates (a common additive). And celery compounds called acetylenics have been shown to stop the growth of tumor cells.

## Pressure Drop

Celery has been used for centuries as a remedy for lowering high blood pressure, and scientists recently discovered why it works: a chemical compound called phthalide helps blood vessels to dilate, which lowers blood pressure. Phthalide also reduces stress hormones, which cause blood vessels to constrict.

Celery's potassium content and its diuretic effect also help prevent and reduce high blood pressure.

## Calm Down

Hippocrates used celery to treat nervous patients, and he was no quack: research has shown that essential oils extracted from celery seed have a tranquilizing effect on the central nervous system.

**Tips:**
Don't neglect to eat the leaves: they contain the most vitamin C, calcium, and potassium. Cooked celery retains its nutrients; try sautéing it lightly to retain its crunch.

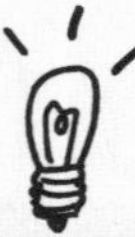

**STREET SMARTS**

"I always believed in the healing power of food as a mental as well as a physical thing," says Kate Pratt, a thirty-eight-year-old book editor. "Eating a bowl of my mother's chicken soup always made me feel better when I was sick—it made me feel cared for. Now I know it's not all in my head—at least in one sense—because I know it really helps my stuffy nose, too. But to me that's secondary."

# Chili Peppers

- Lower cholesterol
- Help prevent blood clots
- Improve circulation
- May help prevent heart disease
- May reduce cancer risk
- Act as decongestants
- May help prevent ulcers

Most people associate chili peppers with super-spicy meals, not super-healthy ones. Maybe you never go near them because you don't enjoy a flaming tongue. If so, you're making a mistake: although chili peppers can be eye-poppingly hot, they are always a great addition to a healing diet.

## A Peck of Nutrients

You're unlikely to eat a heaping serving of chili peppers at one sitting; fortunately, just one contains as much antioxidant protection as it does peppy flavor. One chili contains 100 percent of the RDA for beta-carotene and almost 200 percent of the RDA for vitamin C.

Both beta-carotene and vitamin C help the body fight free radicals that can lead to cell damage and, in turn, to cancer, cholesterol-clogged arteries, and heart disease. These antioxidant vitamins also help fight premature aging and work to strengthen the immune system.

Chili peppers contain a compound called capsaicin, which gives them their heat as well as many of their healing benefits. Capsaicin appears to help reduce dangerous LDL cholesterol and prevent blood clots, both of which are linked to heart disease.

**F.Y.I.**

Drinking a glass of milk will douse the heat of chili peppers because casein, a protein in milk, counters the chili's heat-giving capsaicin.

## Pain Relief

Chilis have been used through the ages to relieve pain, and now there's proof they really work. Researchers have recently found that capsaicin temporarily blocks a chemical that transmits pain signals through the nervous system. It works so well, in fact, that capsaicin ointment is now used to relieve arthritis, psoriasis, and nerve pain. And researchers are testing capsaicin nose spray as a treatment for cluster headaches.

Capsaicin not only soothes pain, but it may also soothe your mind by releasing mood-lifting endorphins into your brain.

### Hot and Hotter

All chili peppers offer antioxidant nutrients, but the hotter varieties give you more capsaicin. The mildest varieties include Spanish pimentos and Anaheim and Hungarian cherry peppers; the hottest include Scotch bonnet and habañero peppers. In between are jalapeños.

**F.Y.I.**

Contrary to popular belief (and many decades of medical advice), chili peppers do not cause ulcers. In fact, they seem to help prevent them, by stimulating the flow of gastric juices that protect the stomach lining, kill bacteria, and promote digestion.

Chili peppers may even help you lose weight! Studies have shown that just a teaspoon of chili sauce can raise your metabolic rate by 25 percent for hours after a meal.

### Cold Comfort

Capsaicin is also responsible for chili peppers' congestion-clearing action. The peppers' heat stimulates secretions that help loosen mucus in your nose and lungs, providing the same relief as many drugstore cold treatments.

**Tips:**
Chili peppers can irritate your face and eyes; be sure to wash your hands after cutting them. Cooking will destroy much of the vitamin C in chili peppers, but it won't affect the beneficial capsaicin. Also, be sure to eat chilis' thin, spongy membrane; it contains much of the capsaicin.

## Mangoes

- Aid digestion
- May help protect against cancer
- May help prevent heart disease and stroke

Mangoes are among the most popular of tropical fruits because they taste so decadently good, not because they're so good for you. A super-healthy way to "have your cake and eat it too," their sweet, juicy flesh packs a nutritional wallop.

### Antioxidant Riches

One mango provides about 1,000 IUs of beta-carotene—more than 150 percent of the RDA. It also contains 95 percent of the RDA for vitamin C. Together these disease-fighting antioxidants do double battle against the free radicals that can damage healthy cells and cause cancer. Antioxidants also help stop free radicals from damaging dangerous LDL cholesterol, making it less likely to stick to artery walls and cause arteriosclerosis, heart attacks, and stroke.

### Fiber Aid

Mangoes offer one of the best, and most digestible, sources of fiber. More than half of it is soluble fiber, the kind that attaches to and removes cholesterol from the body, thereby reducing risk of heart disease. And the insoluble fiber in mangoes helps maintain bowel regularity, causing stools and any harmful substances in them to move quickly through the body, thus reducing risk of colorectal cancer.

**Tips:**
You may need to handle mangoes with kid gloves—or plastic gloves, anyway. Mangoes belong to the same family as poison ivy, and their peel can severely irritate skin. Even if you've never had a reaction before, you may still be susceptible, especially if you handle several mangoes at a time.

Keep mangoes in a cool, dark place to ripen; that helps them retain their vitamin C content.

## Mushrooms

- Strengthen immune system
- Lower cholesterol
- May reduce risk of heart disease
- May help prevent cancer

In Asia, mushrooms are an enduring symbol of longevity, and the Chinese have used them medic-

**F.Y.I.**

So far, the common white button mushroom has not been shown to have the healing properties of Asian mushrooms, such as maitake, oyster, enoki, tree ears, and, especially, shiitake. But it *is* full of B vitamins.

All mushrooms, even the humble white button mushroom, are a great—and rare—vegetable source of B vitamins. Niacin helps your body convert food into energy and keep tissues healthy. Riboflavin is essential to convert other nutrients, such as niacin, and folate, into usable forms. And the vitamin $B_{12}$ in just three button mushrooms is enough to meet the RDA for this nutrient, which is essential for keeping the brain and nerves healthy.

inally for some 6,000 years. But until Americans started developing a taste for more exotic cuisines, the most nutritious types of mushrooms, such as Asian shiitakes and maitakes, were nowhere to be found on supermarket shelves or dinner tables. Fortunately, all that has changed, as shiitakes and their brethren have become immensely popular for their meaty, smoky, hearty goodness. They deserve to be equally popular for their healing goodness.

## Immune Power

Asian mushrooms have potent immunity-building powers. Shiitakes contain a compound called lentinan that revs up the immune system, strengthening the body against infection and disease. Studies have shown that lentinan is even more effective than powerful prescription drugs in fighting influenza and other viruses. It has also been shown to slow the AIDS virus in the body.

Lentinan may offer protection against cancer as well. When fed to lab animals with tumors, lentinan, in the form of dried mushroom powder, inhibited tumor growth by up to 67 percent.

Another Asian mushroom, maitake, contains beta-glucan, a compound that has been shown to reduce tumors; researchers believe it may be even more effective at fighting disease than lentinan.

## Heart Protection

Eating shiitakes is good for your heart. Shiitakes contain a compound called eritadenine that has been shown to reduce cholesterol levels. One study showed that a group of women eating three ounces of shiitakes a day for a week reduced their cholesterol levels by an average of 12 percent. Shiitakes and other Asian mushrooms also appear to thin the blood and help prevent dangerous clots.

**Tips:**
More and more markets now carry Asian mushrooms, particularly the popular shiitakes, but if you don't find the fresh version, dried mushrooms are a convenient and nutritious alternative. To prepare dried mushrooms, put them in a pan and cover them with water. Bring the water to a boil, then simmer for about 20 minutes. Drain the mushrooms and add them to your recipe. You can use the water to make soup stock.

## Oats

- Reduce cholesterol
- Stabilize blood sugar levels
- Ease constipation
- Help control appetite
- Soothe nerves
- May help prevent heart disease and stroke
- May help prevent cancer

Soon after the cholesterol-heart disease link came to light, oat bran was proved to help reduce cholesterol levels. Overnight, oat bran muffins became the rage among health-conscious eaters. Then, like most fads, they disappeared just as quickly—before many people even realized that oats don't have to come in muffins.

Over the years people have become a lot savvier about the cholesterol-nutrition link, and oatmeal and other oat-filled foods have soared in popularity. But many people are still unaware of its many other health benefits.

**F.Y.I.**

The complex carbohydrates and fiber in oats helps stabilize blood sugar levels, which benefits diabetics as well as anyone seeking long-lasting energy.

Oats have long been used to treat nervousness, and recent evidence shows they really do have calming powers. For example, one study of heavy smokers quitting the habit found that withdrawal symptoms were eased more by an oat extract than by a placebo. The complex carbohydrates and fiber in oats probably contribute to this soothing effect; they help steady blood sugar levels and stabilize mood.

## Cholesterol Curers

Unlike most grains, oats are never refined, so all the nutritional goodness of their outer layers—the bran and germ—remains intact. That goodness includes plentiful doses of fiber and antioxidants, which makes oats a potent weapon against cholesterol and heart disease.

Oats launch a many-pronged attack against cholesterol:

- A soluble fiber called beta-glucan traps dietary cholesterol in the intestine and flushes it out of the body.
- Compounds called saponins bind to and eliminate cholesterol and cholesterol-containing bile.
- A number of antioxidant compounds in oats help control oxidation, the process that harms LDL cholesterol and causes it to stick to artery walls, and also act on the liver to reduce cholesterol production. Researchers believe some of these compounds are far more powerful antioxidants than either vitamin C or E.

## Anticancer Power

Vitamin E and other antioxidants in oats also help strengthen the immune system by routing out foreign invaders such as bacteria and cancer cells. Other compounds in oats protect against cancer by neutralizing free radicals before they can cause trouble.

Oats also contain phytic acids, which may help prevent colon cancer by binding to and eliminating dangerous minerals. But phytic acids do have their down side: they can also limit the absorbability of good minerals such as iron, zinc, and calcium from other foods. They're not a problem as long as you don't make eating oats an everyday habit.

**Tips:**
Quick-cooking oats offer the same nutrients as the old-fashioned kind, but contain added sodium.

If you're trying to cut calories, oat bran is a better choice than oatmeal: a cup of bran has 87 calories; a cup of oats has 145. They both contain the same nutrients.

Because they are high in polyunsaturated fat, oats can turn rancid quickly. Store them in an airtight container in a cool, dark place and use them within a few months.

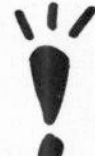

**SMART MOVE**

"As far as I'm concerned, you can take the whole food pyramid and just pour olive oil over it," said an only-half-joking Walter Willet, chairman of the Department of Nutrition at the Harvard School of Public Health, at a conference on the Mediterranean diet.

## Olive Oil

- Lowers dangerous LDL cholesterol
- Helps prevent blood clots
- Lowers blood pressure
- Helps prevent heart disease
- Reduces cancer risk

In Mediterranean countries it's been a top healing food for thousands of years. But in the U.S., olive oil was until recently considered just another fat, no better than butter.

Then scientists began puzzling over the fact that Greece, Spain, southern France, and Italy had unusually low rates of heart disease despite a high fat intake. On closer examination of the Mediterranean diet, they found their solution: people in those countries have a high intake of monounsaturated fat—almost all of it olive oil—whereas the Western diet is high in saturated fat.

Since that discovery, olive oil has undergone a dramatic change of status—from no-no to health necessity.

## More Heart Protection

Researchers have also found that olive oil contains hundreds of chemical compounds that perform heart-protective functions. These compounds provide antioxidant protection against free radical cell damage, thin the blood to prevent clots, lower blood pressure, and prevent absorption of excess cholesterol in the body.

## Anticancer Effects

Olive oil's antioxidant compounds also protect against cancer. Although researchers don't yet know why, olive oil appears to be especially protective against breast cancer; one study found that women who consumed olive oil at least twice a day had a 25 percent lower risk of breast cancer than women who consume it less often.

**Tips:**
Remember that for all its healthy benefits, olive oil is still a fat, and experts recommend keeping your fat intake to 30 percent or less of your daily calories. So don't go overboard.

# Onions

- Lower cholesterol
- Combat infections
- May help prevent cancer
- May help reduce risk of heart disease and stroke
- May help prevent asthma

If you tend to avoid onions on your sandwich for the sake of your breath, read on: once you find out how much onions can do for your health, you may start asking for extra. (And try a sprig or two of parsley to sweeten your breath.)

## Disease-Fighting Flavonoids

Recent research has turned up impressive evidence of onions' healing powers: a large study showed that people who eat more onions in their daily diets have lower rates of stomach cancer.

Another study demonstrated that men who ate a quarter-cup of onions a day, along with four cups of tea and an apple, were one-third less likely to die from heart attacks as those who ate the least amounts of these foods.

Part of the credit for these results goes to antioxidant compounds called flavonoids. Onions contain dozens of these compounds, which have been found to provide strong protection against free radical damage. The main flavonoid found in onions, quercetin, has strong heart-protecting benefits: it helps prevents damaging LDL cholesterol from oxidizing and sticking to artery walls, and it also helps prevent the formation of harmful blood clots. Quercetin also has been shown to halt the growth of tumors in animals. Researchers believe that quercetin and other onion compounds not only stop tumor growth but also kill harmful bacteria that may lead to tumors.

## The Upside of Crying

Onions contain potent sulfur compounds—they're the ones that make you cry as you slice. Researchers believe that these compounds raise levels of good cholesterol, which helps keeps arterial plaque at bay. These sulfur compounds also lower levels of dangerous blood fats called triglyc-

**SMART SOURCES**

These cookbooks are filled with good ideas about food combining and preparing vegetarian meals.

*American Wholefoods Cuisine: 1,300 Meatless, Wholesome Recipes from Short Order to Gourmet*
by Nikki and David Goldbeck

*The New Laurel's Kitchen: A Handbook for Vegetarian Cooking*
by Laurel Robertson, Carol Flinders, and Brian Ruppenthal

**F.Y.I.**

Freshly squeezed OJ is a great drink: it's high in vitamin C, potassium, and folic acid. But don't neglect to eat the whole fruit as well: juice doesn't provide all the fiber and other beneficial compounds.

erides; fewer triglycerides means thinner blood, which in turn means lower blood pressure.

Onions' sulfur compounds are also a boon to asthma sufferers: they help stop allergic reactions and inflammation, helping to clear respiratory passages.

Just one medium onion per day provides all these healthy benefits.

**Tips:**

Cut onions close to cooking or serving time to preserve the most nutrients.

Store onions in the refrigerator or in a cool place. Chilled onions will provoke fewer tears when you cut them; running your knife blade under cold water helps too.

# Oranges

- Strengthen the immune system
- Lower cholesterol
- Prevent inflammation
- May lower risk of heart disease and stroke
- May help prevent cancer

Oranges are a strong contender for most popular fruit and food most associated with good health. Even nutritional know-nothings know oranges are a great source of vitamin C. But few realize how many other good things they do for you.

## C Plus

An average orange contains about 70 milligrams of vitamin C, over 100 percent of the RDA for this powerful antioxidant. Vitamin C helps the body fight cell-damaging free radicals that can lead to cancer, dangerous levels of LDL cholesterol, heart disease, and stroke. It also helps fortify the immune system, warding off infection and spurring the healing process.

But that's not all. Oranges also contain a variety of other compounds that are believed to have even stronger antioxidant powers. Researchers believe that antioxidant flavonoids such as hesperidin may be up to six times as potent as vitamin C in fighting high cholesterol and other disease risk factors. Hesperidin also has been shown to help stop inflammation without irritating the stomach (as aspirin can).

## Cancer Protection

Many studies show that people who eat more oranges and other citrus fruits have lower rates of stomach cancer. Citrus fruits may help prevent nitrates and nitrites, which are found in smoked meats and other foods, from becoming cancer-causing nitrosamines.

Another compound, called limonene, appears to help prevent breast and lung cancers. Researchers believe limonene, which is found in orange and other citrus oils, reduces the growth of tumors and prevents the formation of new tumors.

## Double Dose of Fiber

Oranges are a good source of both soluble and insoluble fibers. Pectin, the soluble fiber that's found mainly in the skin around each orange section and in the peel, helps trap and eliminate cholesterol from the body—especially dangerous LDL cholesterol. Try to eat a little of the white part of the orange peel as well as the fruit; it contains half of the fruit's pectin supply.

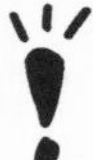

**SMART MOVE**

Michael Janson, M.D., author of *The Vitamin Revolution in Health Care*, says getting copious amounts of vitamin C is crucial in today's polluted world: "We can't breathe clean air, we can't avoid secondhand cigarette smoke, we can't avoid pesticides and other chemicals. Vitamin C helps to detoxify many of these chemicals."

The insoluble fiber in oranges helps prevent and relieve constipation and other digestive problems. By moving potentially toxic substances more quickly through your digestive system, it also helps reduce the risk of colon cancer.

**Tips:**
Orange peel and oil (found in the peel) are as valuable as the flesh. Add orange zest (strands of orange peel) to salads and baked goods to get their benefits. Oranges begin to lose their vitamin C as soon as they are picked, so eat them as soon as possible.

# Peas

- Reduce cholesterol
- Stabilize blood sugar levels
- Can help improve mood, appetite, and sleep
- May help reduce risk of heart disease
- May help prevent cancer

Probably because they've been subjected to the gray, mealy canned peas in high school cafeterias, many people would rate peas low on the taste and nutrition scale. But fresh peas bear no relation to their processed counterparts; delicately delicious, they're also tiny dietary dynamos.

## Meaty Nutrition

Rich in protein and minerals, peas are the vegetable equivalent of liver—without the fat and cholesterol.

A 5-ounce serving of fresh peas gives you a good dose of iron as well as 100 percent of the RDA for thiamin (vitamin $B_1$)—even more than you get from thiamin-rich liver. That's significant because thiamin is often shortchanged in the American diet. The elderly, people under stress, and heavy drinkers are especially liable to have borderline thiamin levels; deficiency can lead to depression, sleeplessness, loss of appetite, and memory problems. Studies indicate that people who ingest higher levels of $B_1$ improve in all these areas.

## Colorful Cancer Fighters

Chlorophyllin, the pigment that makes peas green, does double duty as a cancer preventer. It latches on to cancer-causing free radicals and helps shepherd them out of the body before they can do any cellular damage.

## Fiber-Rich Benefits

Peas provide more than 4 grams of soluble fiber per half-cup serving. Pea fiber is powerful stuff: studies show that it helps reduce levels of triglycerides, a factor in heart disease. It also helps reduce cholesterol, especially the dangerous LDL cholesterol that can lead to arteriosclerosis.

Another benefit: the fiber in peas slows down digestion and stabilizes blood sugar levels, which is particularly helpful to diabetics.

**Tips:**

Garden peas have more thiamin than sugar snap peas or snow peas. All three are good sources of iron and fiber.

Frozen peas retain a high levels of nutrients—canned peas don't. Steam rather than boil peas to retain the most nutrients.

# Red Peppers

- Help prevent eye problems
- May reduce risk of heart disease and stroke
- May help prevent cancer

Part of the capsicum family, which also includes pimento and chili peppers, red peppers are native to the Americas, and have been used for over five thousand years as an important food and medicine source. Modern nutritional science has been a little slow to catch up, but—as is so often the case—there's now impressive evidence to confirm the Native Americans' wisdom.

## Tops in Disease Protection

Among the very best antioxidant sources, red peppers offer an impressive arsenal of nutrients that prevent cancer and protect the heart. They're loaded with vitamin C; one pepper provides 150 percent of the RDA, which is far more than even an orange offers. And the average red pepper has 4,220 IUs of beta-carotene—more than 80 percent of the RDA. Both have been shown to fight the free radical cell damage that can lead to serious disease.

Red peppers are one of the few foods that contain lycopene, a carotenoid that may help to prevent certain kinds of cancer. Recent studies show that people with low levels of lycopene are at greater risk of developing cancers of the cervix, bladder, and pancreas.

## Age Fighters

Together, vitamin C and beta-carotene provide a double dose of protection against the free radical damage that can lead not only to disease but also to wrinkles, cataracts, and other aging problems.

In addition, red peppers supply the phytonutrient compounds lutein and zeaxanthin, both of which have been shown to protect against macular degeneration, the main cause of visual impairment in the elderly.

**Tips:**
To cook or not to cook? You benefit either way. Raw peppers retain the most vitamin C, which is easily destroyed in cooking. But cooking releases beta-carotene from peppers, making it more available to your body. So eat them raw in salads and sandwiches as well as lightly grilled or sautéed.

Eat peppers with a little bit of fat to help your body absorb the most beta-carotene.

Peppers' naturally waxy skin helps protect them from damaging oxidation, so their vitamin content remains intact even after several weeks. Refrigeration keeps them fresh longest.

**F.Y.I.**

For every 1 percent you lower your cholesterol, your risk of heart disease drops 2 percent.

## Red Wine

- Lowers cholesterol
- Helps prevent blood clots
- Fights infection
- May help prevent heart and circulatory disease

Wine has a long history as a healing food: the Jewish Talmud termed it "the foremost of all medicines." But most people consume it for pleasure, not as a preventive measure, and in recent times its health benefits have been largely forgotten. Now that nutritionists have given thumbs up to the wine-friendly Mediterranean diet, wine has

**F.Y.I.**

Although wine does not contain high amounts of iron, what it does have is very well absorbed by the body.

regained its status as a beverage that's delicious and beneficial.

## The Alcohol Factor

Recent research indicates that drinking small amounts of any type of alcoholic beverage helps prevent heart disease. The ethanol, or alcohol, in alcoholic beverages seems to raise levels of heart-protecting HDL cholesterol. But wine's benefits go further than this.

## Why Wine?

Wine is better for you than other kinds of alcohol because it contains a high concentration of flavonoids. Researchers believe these beneficial compounds, including quercetin and resveratrol, may have even more heart-protective effects than vitamin E. Flavonoids help keep dangerous LDL cholesterol from sustaining free radical damage, which can cause them to stick to artery walls. Quercetin also helps prevent harmful blood clots, another factor in heart disease and stroke.

Flavonoids are far more concentrated in red wine than in white. The longer wine ferments, the more flavonoids are released, and red wine ferments much longer than white.

## Infection Protection

Throughout the ages, wine has been used as an antiseptic and disinfectant. No less a bacterial authority than Louis Pasteur called wine "the most healthful and most hygienic of beverages." In the 1800s, scientists found that wine could kill cholera and typhoid germs, a fact once attributed to its alcohol content. But French researchers have discovered that it's the polyphenol compounds in wine that are responsible for destroying bacteria.

Wine fights everyday intestinal germs as well, so a glass with dinner may help prevent traveler's diarrhea and other digestive woes. Grapes or unfermented grape juice won't do as much good: wine's antibacterial properties are fully released during fermentation.

**Tips:**
Health experts recommend that maximum health benefits come from drinking wine in moderation. For women, that's one 5-ounce glass a day; for men, two 5-ounce glasses.

**F.Y.I.**

The healthiest wines are those that contain the most tannin, the substance that makes wine dry. Go for the heartiest wines, such as merlot, cabernet, and port.

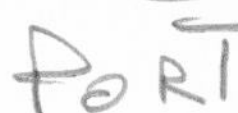

## The Down Side

Wine may contain added preservatives, colors, and flavors that are not listed on the label; some of these may cause adverse reactions. The preservative sulfur dioxide, for example, may trigger asthma in those who are susceptible.

Red wine also causes migraine headaches in some people. Researchers now believe that chemical substances called congeners may be responsible for this problem.

Here's a general rule of thumb: the cheaper the wine, the more chemical additives it will contain. You're better off spending a little more and drinking it conservatively. Buying organic wines may not make much difference, as it is generally the chemicals added during wine production, not those used in growing grapes, that pose the greatest health threat.

You should not drink wine or other alcohol if you have a tendency toward gout. Alcohol is also linked to liver problems, higher blood pressure, heart arrhythmias—and alcoholism. Pregnant women are advised to abstain from all alcoholic beverages, which can cause fetal alcohol syndrome.

Finally, despite the benefits linked to moderate wine drinking, physicians don't recommend consuming alcohol for that reason.

## Rice

- Helps reduce cholesterol
- Maintains the digestive system
- Stabilizes blood sugar levels
- Boosts mood and brain function
- May help prevent heart disease and high blood pressure
- May cut cancer risk

It's hard to believe white rice and brown rice come from the same source.

Processed within an inch of its life, white rice comes to you stripped of almost all its flavor as well as its nutrients—except the ones with which it gets "fortified." Brown rice, on the other hand, is minimally processed; it's the whole grain without the inedible husk. Full of rich flavor and the nutrients nature gave it, brown rice has nearly twice the fiber or of white rice, as well as more vitamins and potassium.

It's not hard to guess which is the better bet.

### What about Wild Rice?

Wild rice is not a rice at all, but the seeds of a freshwater grass. So it would be inaccurate to call it the most nutritious type of rice; but if it were a rice, it would be.

Wild rice contains twice as much protein as true rice, along with more riboflavin, niacin, zinc, and linoleic acid, which helps reduce cholesterol levels. It's got a deliciously nutty, woodsy flavor, too. The only drawback: wild rice is expensive. But when you consider all the benefits, it's well worth adding to your menu at least a couple of times a month; less expensive brown rice–wild rice mixes are now available.

## Bran Matters

Bran, the outer layer of brown rice, contains a compound called orysanol, which helps reduce the body's natural cholesterol production. Studies have shown that people who eat about 3 ounces of rice bran a day for three weeks experience an average 7 percent drop in cholesterol—and an average 10 percent drop in harmful LDL cholesterol, the kind that clogs arteries and ups your risk for high blood pressure, heart disease, and stroke.

## Fiberful

A half cup of brown rice contains about 2 grams of insoluble fiber. In addition to lowering cholesterol, rice bran fiber helps maintain bowel regularity and has been linked to lower risk of bowel cancer. By making potentially dangerous substances move quickly through and out of the body, bran gives toxins less time to damage colon walls and lead to colon cancer.

The fiber in brown rice also binds with excess estrogen in the digestive tract and ushers it out of the body. That means there is less estrogen circulating in the bloodstream, where it may help cause breast cancer.

There's no end to the benefits of fiber: it also helps steady blood sugar levels and provide slow-burning energy, making it good for diabetics and athletes alike.

**Tips:**
Brown basmati rice is the quickest cooking brown rice. When cooking rice, try adding some vegetable or chicken broth to the cooking liquid for a flavor boost. Always let rice cook until all the liquid is absorbed so you won't lose important nutrients.

**F.Y.I.**

Rice is gluten free and unlikely to cause an allergy, so it's a good bet for anyone who is allergic to wheat.

In addition, a 7-ounce serving of brown rice provides about a third of the RDA for thiamin (vitamin $B_1$). Borderline thiamin deficiency is common in whole-grain-deprived American diets, and a lack of thiamin can lead to a host of health problems including depression, irritability, and an inability to concentrate.

Brown rice is filled with oils and will quickly spoil at room temperature. Refrigerate uncooked rice in an airtight container; it will keep for up to a year.

## Salmon

- Helps relieve symptoms of rheumatoid arthritis
- Helps prevent osteoporosis (canned salmon)
- Reduces inflammation
- May reduce risk of heart disease and stroke
- May help prevent cancer

All fish offer a bounty of nutritional benefits, but salmon is a fin or two ahead of the rest. Its high fat content gives salmon a rich, satisfying taste; surprisingly, it also accounts for salmon's outstanding healing properties.

### Heart-Healthy Fat

Salmon is low in calories and cholesterol, but high in the type of fat called omega-3 fatty acids. This is one case in which you can almost say the more fat, the better: omega-3 fatty acids are associated with all kinds of disease-preventing benefits.

Researchers have found that these acids help lower bad LDL cholesterol and triglyceride blood fat in people with elevated levels of these substances, thus reducing the risk of arteriosclerosis, heart attack, and stroke. They appear to work by attacking prostaglandins and other compounds that can cause blood clots and make blood vessels constrict, leading to high blood pressure. They also raise levels of healthy HDL cholesterol, which helps prevent plaque formation in the arteries.

Although it's not yet clear how they do it, omega-3 fatty acids also seem to strengthen the heart muscles and maintain normal heart rhythms. Serious heart irregularities can lead to cardiac arrest.

## Cancer-Fighting Fat

Omega-3 fatty acids have also been shown to slow the growth of cancerous tumors. Here again they work by attacking prostaglandins and other compounds that encourage tumors to grow. The fat seems to work particularly well against breast and colon tumors. Studies have shown that people who include fish in their diets are much less liable to get cancer.

## Canned versus Fresh

Canned and fresh salmon are both great nutritional choices, for slightly different reasons.

Sockeye or red salmon is the type most often sold in cans. Canned salmon eaten with its bones provides 20 percent of the RDA for calcium, as well as vitamin D, which is essential for absorption of calcium.

Coho or Atlantic salmon is sold at fish stores and in restaurants. Any kind of salmon offers a fair amount of fatty fish oil, but Atlantic salmon is by far the best: one 4-ounce serving has 21 grams of omega-3 fatty acids, making it one of the best natural sources of omega-3.

**Tips:**
Salmon is delicious and nutritious whether poached, broiled, or baked. Use canned salmon in salads or in a sandwich on whole-grain bread.

**F.Y.I.**

Eating salmon and other oily fish such as halibut, mackerel, and sardines, has been shown to reduce joint tenderness and pain in rheumatoid arthritis sufferers. It also appears to help prevent ulcerative colitis, a serious condition in which the intestines become inflamed.

In addition, a National Heart and Lung Institute study found that men who ate just 1 gram of omega-3 fatty acids (a fraction of the amount found in salmon) per day could reduce their risk of developing coronary artery disease by up to 40 percent.

**F.Y.I.**

The riboflavin in spinach promotes tissue growth and repair, and helps convert other nutrients into usable form.

Minerals in spinach help regulate the amount of fluid your body retains; proper fluid balance is essential to overall health.

Spinach is a great source of potassium, which helps regulate blood pressure and maintain heart health.

The folic acid in spinach also helps prevent the birth defect spina bifida.

# Spinach

- Helps prevent birth defects
- Helps prevent and treat anemia
- May lower risk of cancer
- May reduce risk of heart disease and stroke
- May cut risk of degenerative eye disease

Leafy green vegetables of all kinds (not including iceberg lettuce) head the list of nutritional bargains; they're full of health-enhancing ingredients and nearly empty of calories. But spinach is near the top of the top of the list. As versatile as it is delicious, it offers an easy way to incorporate more green goodness into your diet.

## Disease Protection

Spinach and other leafy greens are top sources of vitamins C and E and the carotenoids lutein, alpha-carotene, and beta-carotene. All are powerful antioxidants that help neutralize dangerous free radicals and help lower risk of heart disease, strokes, cancer, and cataracts.

Researchers have found that people who eat leafy greens such as spinach are apt to have a lower risk of stomach, skin, prostate, lung, and bladder cancers. For example, a recent study showed that people over age sixty-six who ate the most vegetables rich in carotenes had two-thirds fewer deaths from cancer within the next five years than people who ate the least.

## Toxic Blockers

Spinach's high levels of folic acid and other B vitamins work to keep the body's natural compounds in balance. In particular, they help regulate homocysteine, an amino acid that can become toxic at high levels, contributing to clogged arteries and heart disease. A major study found that people with the highest levels of homocysteine in their blood were three times more likely to have heart attacks than those with lower levels.

## Eye Aid

Age-related macular degeneration (AMD) is the number-one cause of irreversible blindness among American adults. The good news: a recent study found that people who often ate spinach or collard greens were at the lowest risk for AMD—up to 43 percent lower risk, to be exact. Most interestingly, their risk was lower than that of people who ate other carotene-rich foods.

### The Ironic Truth

Thanks to Popeye, even people who know nothing else about nutrition know that spinach is the world's best source of strength-building, anemia-preventing iron. The only problem is, that's not quite true. But neither is it true, as some nutritionists now claim, that it's a lousy source.

Confused? Here's the lowdown. For a long time, it was believed to contain more iron than it actually does. Then researchers discovered that not only was the iron content overestimated, but it was also hard for the body to use, thanks to other compounds called oxalates that interfere with its absorption. So its reputation as an iron provider plummeted.

However, spinach *is* a useful, if not super, source of iron. Studies show that the effects of oxalates may be short-term. In one study, the mineral levels of men who ate one-quarter pound of spinach every other day dropped at first but returned to normal after six weeks.

**F.Y.I.**

Sweet potatoes' high vitamin E levels help boost male fertility.

The potassium in sweet potatoes (one potato provides about half the RDA) also helps prevent high blood pressure and maintains heart health.

Sweet potatoes are also a good source of iron, especially for vegetarians.

**Tips:**
Aim to eat spinach a couple of times a week; more than that and you'll risk consuming too many mineral-inhibiting oxalates. *Warning!* People with gout or kidney or bladder stones should avoid spinach because of its oxalates.

Frozen spinach retains more nutrients than older fresh spinach. Canned spinach retains most nutrients except folic acid.

# Sweet Potatoes

- Help prevent and regulate high blood pressure
- Help prevent and treat anemia
- Help control diabetes
- Help prevent birth defects
- May help prevent cancer
- May reduce risk of heart disease and stroke
- May boost male fertility
- May improve memory

It's a shame that so many people eat sweet potatoes only at Thanksgiving time, dotted with melted mini-marshmallows, glazed with brown sugar and drowned in butter. The unadulterated spud is far more delicious—and needless to say, far more nutritious.

## Disease Fighters

Sweet potatoes are packed with antioxidants, which provide powerful protection against the cell damage that can lead to cancer and other diseases.

The bright orange color tells you sweet potatoes are loaded with beta-carotene; an average (4-ounce) potato contains more than 14 grams' worth.

One sweet potato also supplies an average of 28 milligrams of vitamin C, nearly half the RDA. And sweet potatoes are also the very best low-fat source of vitamin E, providing nearly as much of this nutrient as do fatty nuts and seeds. Vitamin E not only helps fight cancer but also helps maintain heart health.

### Diabetes Aids

Because sweet potatoes are high in complex carbohydrates, they fill you up and can help you control your weight. Controlling weight also helps control diabetes.

Sweet potatoes have lots of fiber—more good news for diabetics. Fiber helps lower blood sugar levels by slowing the rate at which food is converted into glucose and absorbed into the bloodstream, which is helpful for anemics, as well.

**Tips:**
Choose sweet potatoes that have a bright color and are firm and smooth skinned. Baking is the best way to retain sweet potatoes' nutrients. A *little* fat will help you absorb the beta-carotene.

## Tea

- Reduces cholesterol
- Helps prevent tooth decay
- Strengthens the immune system
- May help prevent heart disease and stroke
- May reduce risk of cancer

Tea leads a double life. For Americans, it's long been a cheap, convenient drink that's both sooth-

**F.Y.I.**

Recent research supports the traditional use of tea to fight flu. Tea's antioxidants help strengthen the immune system, enabling it to fight flu and other viruses.

Tea is also high in cavity-fighting fluoride. Japanese researchers have also found that four compounds in tea—tannin, catechin, caffeine, and tocopherol—help make tooth enamel resistant to decay.

ing and stimulating—nothing more. Yet there's another reason people the world over drink more tea than any other beverage: the lowly tea leaf has potent health-enhancing powers. The Chinese have known this for some four thousand years; finally, modern research is catching up.

## Serious Medicine

Black and green teas are loaded with flavonoids called polyphenols. Polyphenols act as antioxidants, helping to prevent the free-radical cell damage that leads to cancer, high cholesterol, heart disease, and other serious afflictions.

Researchers studying thirty-nine different antioxidants in foods have found that the polyphenols found in tea are the most potent free-radical fighters of all.

Tea has been shown to reduce tumor formation and is linked to lower levels of skin, breast, lung, esophageal, pancreatic, colon, liver, small intestine, and stomach cancer.

In a study of eight hundred men, those who ate the most flavonoids, including polyphenols, had a 58 percent lower risk of dying from heart disease than those who ate the least. And the healthiest men were those who got more than half their flavonoids from about four cups of black tea a day.

**Tips:**

Steep tea for three minutes to get all the beneficial compounds. Steeping longer will produce more compounds, but it also makes them bitter.

Opt for tea bags rather than loose tea: tea in bags has more polyphenol.

Both green and black teas (regular and decaffeinated) contain health-promoting substances; so do bottled iced tea and powdered tea mixes. But herbal tea doesn't contain leaves from the tea plant, *Camellia sinesis,* so it shares none of the benefits of the others.

## Tofu and Other Soy Foods

- Maintain intestinal health
- Relieve constipation
- Stabilize blood sugar levels
- Can help reduce menopause symptoms
- May help lower risk of heart disease
- May reduce risk of breast and prostate cancer

In Asian countries, soy products are an everyday staple. The Japanese, who eat about 24 pounds of soy food per person per year (Americans eat about 4 pounds), live longer than people anywhere else in the world and have the lowest rates of heart disease. Although no one can say for sure that soy plays a role in these statistics, there's strong evidence in its favor.

### The Healthiest Protein

A 3-ounce serving of tofu provides 20 grams of protein, along with about half the RDA for bone-building calcium and 13 milligrams of iron—that's 87 percent of the RDA for women and 130 percent of the RDA for men. The high iron content in soy foods is absorbed well, unlike that in most plant foods. And although tofu and other soy foods are moderately high in fat, most of the fat is polyunsaturated. All these factors make soy a terrific meat replacer.

Even if you already eat a low-fat diet, you can substantially lower your blood cholesterol by replacing some low-fat animal protein with soy products. Studies have shown that people with raised blood cholesterol levels who ate soy products instead of half or all of the animal protein in their diet, reduced their blood cholesterol by 8 to 16 percent in a few weeks. Researchers attribute this to the particular balance of fiber, fatty acids, and phytoestrogens in soybeans, which help deactivate and remove dangerous LDL cholesterol from the body. Soybeans also contain alpha-linolenic acid, an omega-3 fatty acid linked to improved heart health.

## High-Fiber Benefits

Soybeans, tofu, tempeh, and other soy products are rich in both soluble and insoluble fibers. Soy fiber improves digestion and can prevent and ease constipation, thereby reducing the risk of colon cancer and other bowel diseases.

Soy fiber also helps regulate blood sugar levels. By slowing down the speed of digestion and absorption, fiber fosters a steadier rise and fall of blood sugar, which benefits diabetics and stabilizes energy levels.

## Women and Soy

Early evidence shows that eating soy products reduces hot flashes and other symptoms of menopause and postmenopause, such as loss of bone minerals. Researchers believe this is due to soybeans' high phytoestrogen content.

Soybeans are the richest known source of the phytoestrogen compounds genistein and daidzein, which are weaker versions of the estrogen women produce naturally. When estrogen rises to dangerous levels in the body, phytoestrogens may supplant some of it in the body, helping to return it to normal, safe levels.

Soy has such beneficial effects that researchers foresee a day when it will replace or supplement estrogen replacement therapy.

The phytoestrogens in soy have also been linked to reduced rates of breast cancer. High estro-

## Soy Options

**Tofu.** Made from curdled soy milk, which may not sound too appetizing, tofu is in fact not sour but bland. Its greatest attribute, other than its high nutritional content, is its ability to take on the flavor of other ingredients and seasonings. You can add it to stir-fries, marinate it and use it in place of meat, or even use it to make nondairy versions of desserts such as cheesecake. Firm tofu is highest in calcium (since it's made with the setting compound calcium chloride); the softer types are excellent for making creamy salad dressings.

**Tempeh.** Unlike its bland sibling tofu, tempeh is made from fermented soybeans, which gives it a deep, smoky flavor. It makes a great meat substitute, whether grilled or added to stews, casseroles, or pasta sauces.

**Soy Milk.** Popular with vegetarians and the lactose-intolerant, soy milk is made from ground soybeans and water and has a thicker, creamier consistency than regular milk. It comes in a variety of flavors as well as a reduced-fat version (which may not contain as many beneficial phytoestrogens).

**Soy Flour.** A nutritious substitute for wheat flour, soy flour is made from ground roasted soybeans. Opt for the defatted version, which contains more protein and less fat.

**Texturized Soy Protein.** This is a versatile meat substitute made from soy flour; although you won't mistake it for steak, it works well in seasoned dishes such as casseroles and makes a good "veggie burger."

gen levels are one risk factor for breast cancer; eating foods high in fiber and estrogen-supplanting phytoestrogens helps reduce blood estrogen. One study showed that premenopausal women who consumed high amounts of soy foods, along with beta-carotene and polyunsaturated fats, had only half as much risk of developing breast cancer as women who consumed high amounts of animal protein.

## Men and Soy

Soy may do wonders for men as well. A diet abundant in soy-rich foods seems to help reduce levels of the male hormone testosterone, which may spur the growth of cancerous cells in the prostate gland.

**Tips:**
Raw soybeans, including soybean sprouts, contain a toxin that must be destroyed by thorough cooking before eating. Soak soybeans for at least five hours before cooking, then boil them in fresh water for at least two hours.

When cooking with tofu or other soy products, add them at the end of cooking time. Cooking soy products at high temperatures for extended periods may destroy some of the nutrients. Miso, soy sauce, and soybean oil lack the benefits of other soy products.

You're best off buying full-fat soy products, such as soy milk, because they contain much higher amounts of beneficial phytoestrogens.

Soy milk contains phytoestrogens but little fiber or calcium.

# Tomatoes

- Help prevent cataracts and other age-related ailments
- May help prevent cancer
- May reduce risk of heart disease and stroke

Central to the famously healthy Mediterranean diet, tomatoes are also central to the less famous, less healthy American diet. Americans eat more tomatoes than any other fruit or vegetable—and that's one part of our diet that definitely shouldn't change.

## Life-Enhancing Lycopene

Tomatoes are one of the few fruits and vegetables (by the way, they *are* fruits, not vegetables) that contain the carotenoid called lycopene. Recent research show that lycopene, the pigment that makes tomatoes red, is an antioxidant that helps prevent free radicals from causing cell damage. Researchers now believe that lycopene, which is found both in raw and processed tomatoes, may have twice the antioxidant power of beta-carotene.

Studies indicate that people with the highest levels of lycopene are at much lower risk for developing various forms of cancer including cancer of the bladder, cervix, and pancreas. It has also been found to inhibit colon, rectal, stomach, prostate, breast, lung, and endometrial cancer. One study, conducted at Harvard University, found that men who ate at least ten one-half cup servings of tomatoes per week—raw, cooked, or as a sauce—cut their risk of developing prostate cancer by 45 percent.

On top of that, research also indicates that lycopene may help older people stay active longer.

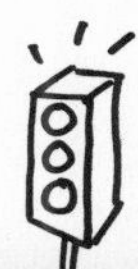

**WHAT MATTERS, WHAT DOESN'T**

### What Matters

- Cooking vegetables briefly so that they retain most of their nutrients.
- Cooking in minimal amounts of water.
- Saving cooking water to use for soups or to sauté other vegetables.

### What Doesn't

- Eating all or most vegetables raw, unless you want to: light cooking can help release nutrients and increases digestibility.

**F.Y.I.**

If you have rheumatoid arthritis, you should avoid tomatoes and other members of the nightshade family (such as potatoes and eggplant), which may worsen this condition.

## More Cancer-Fighting Compounds

Tomatoes also contain coumaric acid and chlorogenic acid, two compounds that may help block the effects of cancer-causing substances called nitrosamines. Nitrosamines form naturally in the body and are also the most lethal carcinogen in tobacco smoke. Coumaric and chlorogenic acids are also found in other fruits and vegetables, and researchers think they may be a major reason that people who eat more produce are less likely to develop cancer.

## Old-Guard Antioxidants

Tomatoes contain substantial levels of more familiar antioxidants, particularly vitamin E, vitamin C, beta-carotene, and the flavonoid quercetin. In addition to lowering the risk of cancer, these nutrients are linked to lower risk of heart disease, stroke, cataracts and other age-related problems.

**Tips:**
By cooking tomatoes you release more of the beneficial compound lycopene. If you cook them in a little olive oil, you'll absorb the lycopene even better.

Canned tomatoes have many of the same nutrients as fresh, but they contain lower levels of vitamin C and carotenes. Tomato paste and sundried tomatoes have plentiful carotenes and vitamin E. Beware of tomato juice: the sodium cancels out the value of tomatoes' potassium.

# Watercress

- Helps prevent and treat infection
- Helps prevent and treat anemia
- Helps protect against birth defects
- Decreases risk of cataracts
- Helps slow effects of aging
- May reduce cancer risk
- May protect against heart disease

With its lively, springlike taste, watercress perks up your tastebuds as well as your diet. It's packed with health-enhancing antioxidants, minerals, and other cruciferous delights.

## Antioxidant Action

Studies show that people who often eat leafy greens, especially cruciferous vegetables such as watercress, have lower rates of cancer. And watercress is particularly beneficial because it's often eaten raw, retaining all its nutrients.

Watercress is high in antioxidants beta-carotene and vitamin C, both linked to lower cancer rates. Researchers believe that it may be especially good at fighting lung cancer caused by smoking or breathing secondhand smoke thanks to a natural compound called phenethyl isothiocyanate (PEITC).

When lab animals were fed watercress after being exposed to tobacco's cancer-causing chemicals, they were 50 percent less likely to develop cancer than animals who got the same chemicals but no watercress. And researchers have found similar results in people who smoke. That's not to say that watercress can delete, or even significantly diminish, the lethal effects of cigarette smoke. But it does appear to have a powerful cancer-fighting effect.

**F.Y.I.**

The rich folic acid content of watercress helps prevent anemia as well as the birth defect spina bifida.

Watercress is also a good source of bone-strengthening calcium; your body can absorb this mineral almost as well from watercress as from milk.

The antioxidant workers in watercress are also believed to help lower cholesterol and prevent heart disease and stroke. Age-related problems such as cataracts and wrinkles may also be slowed by the antioxidants beta-carotene and vitamin C.

## Infection Prevention

Watercress has long been used to fight infection, and with good reason: its vitamin C, zinc, and folic acid all enhance immune system function and have antibiotic effects. The mustard oil in watercress also stimulates circulation and production of gastric acid, which sterilizes bacteria in food.

**Tips:**
Watercress can be stored for about two days in the refrigerator. Keep it in a plastic bag or refrigerate stems in a glass of water.

Watercress is most nutritious when eaten raw. It's also delicious lightly sautéed with garlic; but beware that it loses its ability to release PEITC when cooked.

# Wheat Germ

- Improves digestion and prevents and relieves constipation
- Helps prevent birth defects
- May reduce risk of heart disease
- May help prevent cancer

Wheat germ, the most nutrient-rich part of wheat, offers a plethora of benefits with every sprinkle—proof that good things do indeed come in small packages.

Above all, it's a valuable source of vitamin E. Most of the vitamin E in wheat is concentrated in the germ layer. Getting even the RDA for vitamin E—which many experts consider an insufficient amount—from food sources can be tough; but one ounce of wheat germ oil provides almost 40 milligrams of the vitamin, close to the 40 to 60 milligrams recommended by many for high antioxidant protection.

## Vitamin E Power

A high vitamin E intake is strongly linked to lower risk of heart disease and stroke. Researchers believe this antioxidant may play a direct role in lowering blood cholesterol levels and preventing arteriosclerosis. Experts also theorize that the vitamin E in wheat causes the liver to produce less natural cholesterol.

Research backs up these theories: in one study, people with high cholesterol were given 20 grams (about a quarter cup) of wheat germ a day for four weeks. For the next fourteen weeks, they were given 30 grams. At the end of the study, cholesterol levels had dropped by an average of 7 percent.

Vitamin E is also closely linked to decreased cancer risk. It helps block free radicals and also stimulates the immune system. It even helps prevent the formation of cancer-causing compounds.

## Fiber Action

Vitamin E has a cancer and heart-disease fighting ally in fiber. Three tablespoons of wheat germ provide 3.9 grams of fiber, more than twice as much as a serving slice of whole wheat bread. Because fiber helps ease constipation, it assists in moving poten-

**F.Y.I.**

Folic acid, which is abundant in wheat germ, may help protect against cervical and other cancers and is essential to reducing the risk of having a baby with the birth defect spina bifida.

tially dangerous substances through the colon more quickly and thus helps reduce colon cancer risk. Together with vitamin E it may be effective against many other cancers as well. Fiber is also a great digestive aid.

**Tips:**
What germ is high in phytic acid, which reduces absorption of its high iron and zinc content. Eat a vitamin C–rich food at the same meal to increase absorption.

Because it contains lots of oils, wheat germ can spoil easily; always keep it refrigerated. Do the same with wheat germ oil. Don't eat either one if it starts tasting bitter rather than sweet.

# Yogurt

- Strengthens immune system
- Helps prevent gastrointestinal, yeast, and urinary tract infections
- Helps cure diarrhea
- Helps prevent and heal ulcers
- Helps prevent osteoporosis

Yogurt has a longstanding reputation as a life-enhancing and life-extending food. Though no one's ever proved it can help you live to age 120, there is plenty of evidence that it can help make your years healthy ones.

## Infection Protection

The live *Lactobacillus acidophilus* cultures in yogurt are largely responsible for the power of yogurt to prevent infection. A traditional cure for vaginal yeast infections, its efficacy has now been scientifically validated: a recent study showed that women who ate 8 ounces of yogurt a day had significantly fewer yeast infections than those who did not. *Lactobacillus acidophilus* have been shown to help prevent and treat gastrointestinal and urinary tract infections as well.

## Immune System Strength

Yogurt's *Lactobacillus acidophilus* cultures may also help ward off other infections by stimulating body cells that fight bacteria. According to another study, people who ate two 8-ounce servings of live-culture-containing yogurt a day had higher blood levels of gamma-interferon, a substance that helps the body fight disease. The yogurt eaters also had 25 percent fewer colds and fewer symptoms of hay fever and allergy than nonyogurt eaters.

Yogurt also speeds recovery from diarrhea. Its beneficial cultures work to overcome the "bad" bacteria, such as *E. coli*, which is famous for causing diarrhea in children and travelers alike. Yogurt's antibacterial action restores microbial balance, and thus normal digestive activity.

Yogurt works the same way against ulcers. Yogurt's beneficial bacteria act like antibiotics in the digestive tract, doing battle with the harmful bacteria that cause ulcers, making it difficult for the germs to continue doing harm. Yogurt also contains lactose, a natural sugar that breaks down into lactic acid and helps restore your digestive system to normal.

## Osteoporosis Prevention

Plain, low-fat yogurt is a great source of calcium; one cup contains about 40 percent of the RDA. Cal-

**F.Y.I.**

Yogurt is also a good source of potassium, which helps maintain normal heart function and blood pressure; riboflavin, which is essential for converting food to energy; and vitamin $B_{12}$, which works with folic acid to prevent anemia.

cium is essential in helping prevent osteoporosis, the bone-weakening disease that afflicts many older women in particular. Yogurt's a particularly good choice for people who are unable to digest milk.

**Tips:**
Read yogurt labels carefully: opt for low-fat or nonfat types, and be sure they contain *Lactobacillus acidophilus.* Try to buy yogurt that's less than a week old; it suffers a precipitous loss of live cultures after it's been sitting on the shelf for a while.

Frozen yogurt doesn't offer remotely as many nutrients as regular yogurt. Low-fat or nonfat frozen yogurt is still better than ice cream, though.

***THE BOTTOM LINE***

A top foods list can't possibly encompass all the foods that enhance good health. Reach for these nutritional powerhouses often, but don't reach for them exclusively: for every food in this list, there are several others that provide similar healing benefits, as the following chapter will attest.

CHAPTER 4

# Other Healthy Favorites

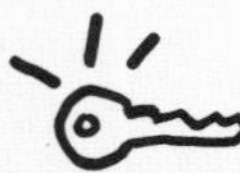

**THE KEYS**

- Don't get in a diet rut: variety means better health.
- There's a bounty of healing foods that belong on your weekly shopping list.
- Question your assumptions about foods you thought you should avoid—but which have many benefits.
- Learn the whys behind what you should eat: here's a rundown of healing nutrients in each food.
- Try out more healing recipes to expand your culinary and nutritional horizons.

Variety is the spice of life: it's a tired cliché, but one that takes on new meaning when applied to the foods you eat. Many people associate healthy eating with proscriptive diets, the kind that tell you exactly what you can and cannot eat. The list of "good" foods is usually so limited that you're bound to raid the "bad" list sooner or later.

But not only is this way of eating self-defeating; it's also unhealthy. A truly healthy diet is one that encompasses a wide range of delicious and nutritious foods. Fortunately, nature provides enough of these that you need never get bored. More importantly for your health, eating many different types of foods vastly improves the chances that you'll get all the nutrients—both known and yet-to-be-discovered—that your body needs to prevent and fight disease and keep you functioning at your peak.

So although the twenty-nine foods described in chapter 3 are true nutritional powerhouses, you shouldn't limit yourself to those or any other twenty-nine items. This chapter is filled with more worthwhile candidates for your list of dietary "staples"; incorporate them into your menus for a lifetime of always delicious, never dull, dining.

## Fruit

You really can't go wrong eating any type of fruit; they all offer nutritional benefits, along with sweet, delicious flavor that makes it easy to forgo empty-calorie candy and other desserts. But some fruits are more health-packed than others. Following are some top choices for vitamins, minerals, and other healing essentials.

## Avocados

Avocados (yes, they are fruit) are high in fat and calories, but they're still a nutritional bargain. First of all, their fat is mostly the good, monounsaturated kind, and like olive oil, it's rich in antioxidant oleic acid, which helps lower dangerous LDL cholesterol while raising levels of beneficial HDL cholesterol.

Avocados are a very good source of vitamin E and an excellent source of potassium, which helps regulate blood pressure. They're very high in fiber, and contain folic acid and vitamin $B_6$. Certain chemicals in avocados stimulate production of collagen, which makes it great for the skin and explains why you can find it in soap form in the skincare aisle. Opt for the fruit instead: it's not only better for your skin, it's also one of the most delicious foods you can eat.

## Blueberries

These small, unassuming berries are an amazing source of fiber and nutrients. Blueberries are high in the soluble fiber pectin, which has been shown to lower cholesterol and prevent bile acid from being transformed into a more dangerous, potentially cancer-causing form. Their insoluble fiber helps prevent and relieve constipation. Blueberries contain the same compound found in cranberries that curtails urinary tract infections. The anthocyanoside compounds in blueberries help cure diarrhea.

Anthocyanosides are also antioxidants and help fight infection and inflammation. Blueberries are bursting with other antioxidants as well. Ellagic acid appears to prevent cellular damage that can lead to cancer. Wild blueberry flavonoids strengthen blood capillaries and improve circula-

**F.Y.I.**

Researchers have found that a glass of cranberry juice a day is ten times as effective at killing bacteria as conventional antibiotics.

If you opt for cranberry juice, look for the unsweetened, 100 percent natural kind; it's available in natural food stores.

tion. Among its many other benefits, the vitamin C in blueberries helps fight cataracts. Finally, blueberries are a good source of potassium, which helps maintain normal fluid balance, blood pressure, and heartbeat.

## Cantaloupe

Half a cantaloupe gives you a boatload of the antioxidants that help fight cancer, heart disease, and premature aging: it contains more than the RDA for beta-carotene, as well as nearly double the RDA for vitamin C. Cantaloupe's high C content helps the body produce collagen, which is vital for skin and tissue repair.

Cantaloupe also offers more potassium than the famously potassium-rich banana. The potassium in cantaloupe helps eliminate excess sodium, which can cause blood pressure to rise; it may keep plaque from sticking to artery walls, another cause of high blood pressure and heart disease; and it helps flush dangerous LDL cholesterol from the body.

## Cranberries

Cranberries are most famous as a now-proven folk remedy for cystitis, the painful urinary tract infection that afflicts many women. Cranberries' antiviral and antifungal properties also strengthen the immune system against other bacterial attacks. The berries are a good source of antioxidant vitamin C and fiber as well.

## Dates

Dates are rich in fiber, niacin, and potassium. They also contain iron. They're a great energy source, as many desert-hiking Bedouins can attest, and pureed dates are a nutritious substitute for white sugar in baked goods. In the Middle East, dates are considered a sexual stimulant, though research has yet to validate this claim.

## Figs

Out of the context of Fig Newtons (not a healing food, though far from the worst cookie you can eat), many people rarely, if ever, consume figs, either fresh or dried. That's a shame, because they are a wonderful, and wonderful tasting, source of energy and easily digested nutrients. Figs contain beta-carotene, vitamin $B_6$, and potassium. They're also loaded with beneficial soluble and insoluble fibers.

For centuries, figs have been used to treat cancer, and now research shows they really are effective: a fig compound called benzaldehyde has been found to help shrink cancerous tumors. Figs also contain an enzyme called ficin that aids digestion and appears to kill bacteria.

## Grapefruit

One grapefruit supplies about 60 percent of the RDA for vitamin C, but the antioxidant power doesn't end there: grapefruit also contains beta-carotene and lycopene (found in red and pink grapefruit), as well as flavonoids, all of which may protect against bladder, cervical, and pancreatic cancers.

Grapefruit also contains the citrus oil limonene, which has been shown to help stop tumor growth and inhibit the formation of new tumors. Pectin, the soluble fiber in the pith, is an excellent heart protector.

**F.Y.I.**

You'll get far more benefits from peeling and eating a grapefruit like an orange than by sectioning it with a grapefruit knife. The outer part of each section, the pith, contains the bulk of beneficial pectin and bioflavonoids.

## Guavas

These luscious tropical fruits are very rich in antioxidant vitamin C: one provides almost 300 percent of the RDA. They also contain an abundance of soluble fiber as well as beta-carotene, potassium, phosphorus, and calcium, all for very few calories.

## Kiwis

Kiwis deserve to be liberated from the fruit salad and stand on their own as a top healing food. The gem-like green flesh of one kiwi contains 120 percent of the RDA for vitamin C—almost twice as much as an orange. And unlike many fruits and vegetables, which lose many of their nutrients when stored for more than a few days, kiwis retain 90 percent of their vitamin C even after six months, making them a valuable staple for your refrigerator's fruit bin. Kiwis also provide an abundance of heart-protective potassium, more fiber than an apple, and an enzyme called atinidin, which aids digestion. All that for very few calories and an abundance of flavor.

## Lemons and Limes

Both of these citrus fruits are excellent sources of vitamin C, along with B vitamins, vitamin E, potassium, magnesium, calcium, phosphorus, copper, zinc, iron, and manganese. They're also full of bioflavonoids, which act as powerful antioxidants and regulate enzymes that may promote tumor growth; the citrus oil limonene has also been shown to help prevent tumor growth. Terpenes help regulate cholesterol and act as antioxidants, guarding cells against toxic damage. Of course, you're not likely to sit down to a plate of lemons, but every squeeze adds valuable nutrients to vegetables, fruit salads, fish, and beverages.

## Papayas

Like most other orange fruit and vegetables, papayas are an excellent source of the protective antioxidant beta-carotene. They also contain many other beneficial carotenoids; in fact, when researchers rated thirty-nine foods according to carotenoid content, papayas came in at number one. On top of that, they offer more than 300 percent of the RDA for vitamin C, along with plenty of fiber and potassium.

The protease enzymes in papaya, such as papain, are similar to enzymes produced naturally in the stomach and help prevent indigestion. Preliminary studies also indicate that papain may help prevent ulcers and counteract the irritating effects of aspirin and other drugs.

## Peaches

Peaches and their close relatives, nectarines, are a good source of vitamin C and also provide useful amounts of beta-carotene and fiber. Dried peaches, which are much higher in calories, are also higher in nutrients: a 3½-ounce serving provides about 100 percent of the RDA for iron, plus a hefty dose of potassium, carotenes, and niacin.

## Pineapples

A good source of vitamin C, pineapples also provide potassium and manganese, both essential to maintaining tissue health. Pineapples are even more valuable as a source of bromelain enzymes, which aid digestion by breaking down protein, and

**F.Y.I.**

Avoid canned peaches; they lose almost all their vitamin C in processing and are often canned in heavy, sugary syrup.

**F.Y.I.**

***Pineapples***

Be sure to eat fresh, uncooked pineapple for optimal benefits.

At the store, choose fruit that's large and sweet smelling; pineapple stops ripening as soon as it's picked.

***Prunes***

Prunes are often treated with sulfur and coated with mineral oil to keep them soft; those oils can interfere with the body's absorption of fat-soluble vitamins and can harm the lining of the bowel. Rinse nonorganic prunes in warm water before using.

help prevent inflammation and swelling by blocking prostaglandins that cause swelling. Researchers have found that bromelain enzymes can speed recovery from ulcers, injuries, arthritis, surgery, and other problems involving swelling and tissue damage. Pineapple enzymes also help prevent blood clots and may help improve circulation.

## Prunes

Their reputation as constipation curers is well earned: prunes contain hydroxyphenylisatin, a chemical that stimulates the bowel muscles and works as a very gentle laxative. Prunes are an excellent source of soluble fiber, which also helps prevent constipation and, in turn, helps reduce cancer (particularly colon cancer) risk. Prunes have heart-protecting value as well. Their soluble fiber helps reduce levels of plaque-producing LDL cholesterol, and their high potassium content regulates blood pressure. Prunes are rich in iron and contain good amounts of niacin, beta-carotene, and vitamin $B_6$, along with copper and boron—making them essential for regular as well as irregular times.

## Strawberries

These favorite berries are not only delicious but are also bursting with vitamin C: one cup contains 120 percent of the RDA for this antioxidant nutrient. They also contain ellagic acid, another antioxidant that's been shown to prevent carcinogens from attacking healthy cells and turning them cancerous. Strawberries provide iron, an anemia- and fatigue-fighting mineral that's well absorbed thanks to the berries' high C content. Plus they're packed with pectin, the soluble fiber that helps eliminate cholesterol from the body. Because strawberries act as a diuretic, they help ease the joint swelling that occurs with rheumatoid arthritis and gout.

**F.Y.I.**

If you are looking for vitamin C, make sure you eat fresh artichokes; canned or frozen lose a lot of the nutrient during processing.

For folate, go with frozen artichokes; they provide even more of this nutrient than do fresh artichokes.

## Vegetables

As with fruits, you really can't go wrong no matter what vegetable you choose—what matters most to your health is eating as many as possible, and opting for the freshest you can find. (Remember, though, that frozen vegetables often retain more nutrients than "fresh" ones that have sat around for a few days.) Here are some more of the best picks.

### Artichokes

Don't confuse globe artichokes with Jerusalem artichokes, which contain plentiful potassium but few other nutrients. Globe artichokes, on the other hand, are loaded with benefits; just be sure you don't choke them in melted butter (opt for lemon juice instead). One chemical compound in artichokes, called cynarine, stimulates the production of bile and aids digestion. Researchers believe it also helps lower cholesterol and reduce blood pressure. Another compound, silymarin, has been found to act as a potent antioxidant. Lab studies show that it helps prevent skin cancer in lab animals, and is likely to help prevent many other forms of cancer as well; in fact, European practitioners have long used silymarin extract to treat liver cancer.

Artichokes are an excellent source of dietary fiber; a medium artichoke provides about a quarter of your daily requirement. They also provide vitamin C, magnesium, and folic acid, a B vitamin

**F.Y.I.**

***Beets***

Beets are high in oxalates, which have been linked to the formation of kidney stones; if you are susceptible to this condition, you should be careful not to overdo it on beets.

***Brussels Sprouts***

Cruciferous vegetables reduce iodine absorption, so make sure you eat iodine-rich foods if you consume lots of Brussels sprouts.

that's not only essential to prevent certain birth defects and to maintain nerve function, but is also linked to lower rates of heart disease and cancer.

## Asparagus

The active compound in asparagus, called asparagine, has a strong diuretic effect, which is why herbalists have long used asparagus to treat rheumatoid arthritis and other problems involving swelling. The ancient Greeks used it to treat kidney and liver problems. Asparagus is also a good choice if you suffer from PMS-related bloating, and is a top source of glutathione. It contains two other antioxidants as well: folic acid and vitamin E. All three are associated with reduced risk of cancer, heart disease, and age-related degenerative diseases.

## Beets

Beets get their deep ruby color from betacyanin, a compound that appears to deter tumor growth. Long used in Europe to treat cancer, beet juice has been shown to prevent cell mutations that lead to cancer. Beets also contain plenty of folic acid, the antioxidant B vitamin that maintains tissue health; may help prevent heart disease and cancer; and may dramatically reduce the risk of certain birth defects.

Beet greens provide even more of certain nutrients: they're rich in folic acid, potassium, beta-carotene, and vitamin C; they also contain some iron.

## Brussels Sprouts

They look and taste like miniature cabbages, and Brussels sprouts share many of the same nutritional benefits. Like other cruciferous vegetables, they are rich in antioxidant vitamins, including vitamin C (one cup has more than 100 percent of the RDA), vitamin E, and carotenes. They're also packed with cancer-fighting phytonutrients, including indoles, which deactivate estrogens that can trigger tumor growth. Researchers believe that indoles may be particularly effective against breast, colon, and prostate cancers. And sulforaphane, which stimulates cells to produce cancer-fighting enzymes and eliminate toxic waste.

Brussels sprouts are among the top vegetable sources of fiber, with 7.5 grams per one-cup serving—about equal to four slices of whole-grain bread. They also contain plentiful amounts of folic acid, along with potassium and iron.

## Cauliflower

One of the cancer-fighting cruciferous vegetables, cauliflower has fewer nutrients than cabbage and other crucifers but still packs plenty of healing power. First off, it's a good source of antioxidants vitamin C—three cauliflower florets supply more vitamin C than a tangerine—and folic acid. Cauliflower also provides two powerful phytonutrients, sulfurophane and indoles. Sulfurophane spurs production of enzymes that help remove toxins from the body; indoles help reduce harmful levels of estrogen that can lead to breast and prostate cancer.

## Collard Greens

Another cruciferous vegetable, collard greens are full of indoles, the phytonutrients that protect against hormone-related cancers including breast, ovary, testicular, and prostate cancer. Research suggests that eating plenty of collard greens and other crucifers may cut your risk of such cancers in *half.*

**F.Y.I.**

Buy corn at its peak of maturity, when the kernels are juicy and plump; that's when it's most nutritious.

To retain the most nutrients, steam rather than boil corn.

Collard greens are also one of the best low-calorie sources of vitamins and minerals. They're high in folic acid and also supply vitamin $B_6$, both important to regulating blood levels of homocysteine. Studies have shown that people with elevated homocysteine levels are three times likelier to have heart attacks than those with normal levels. Collard greens are high in antioxidant carotenoids, iron, and potassium. They contain calcium, but because collard greens are high in calcium-blocking oxalates, look to other foods for this nutrient.

## Corn

Here's one vegetable that many Americans do eat enough of, and that's a very good thing. Corn is high in protease inhibitors, which have been shown to prevent cancer in lab studies. In fact, researchers have found a strong correlation between corn consumption and low death rates from colon, breast, prostate cancer, and heart disease. Corn's a good source of protein and simple and complex carbohydrates, which provide both short- and long-term energy. An ear of white corn also contains four grams of soluble fiber; yellow corn contains half as much. Both kinds offer plentiful thiamin, the B vitamin that's essential for converting food to energy.

### Corn Oil: Friend or Foe?

Corn oil is high in polyunsaturated fat and has long been known to lower cholesterol better than other vegetable oils. However, unlike olive oil, it also lowers levels of "good" HDL cholesterol, and so is not considered as good a heart-protective choice.

## Eggplant

Eggplant is a member of the healthful *solanaceae* family, along with tomatoes and peppers; all three contain terpenes, phytonutrients that may help deactivate hormones that can cause tumors and may prevent free radicals from damaging healthy cells. Eggplant appears to help reduce plaque buildup in the arteries, which can lead to atherosclerosis and heart disease. The potassium in eggplant also protects the heart by regulating blood pressure and heartbeat.

## Fennel

The seeds and leaves of fennel are used as herbs (see chapter 5); the slightly licorice-like bulb is used in salads and stir-fried dishes. Fennel bulb helps digestion and can help ease intestinal cramps. It also contains compounds that mimic estrogen in the body; researchers believe these compounds may ease menopause symptoms and help prevent estrogen-related cancers such as breast and prostate cancer. And fennel is rich in potassium, which helps prevent and reduce high blood pressure.

## Kale

Kale, like other cruciferous vegetables, is loaded with compounds such as sulforaphane—which stimulates the body to produce cancer-fighting enzymes—and indoles, which deactivate potent estrogens that can stimulate tumor growth.

Kale is an excellent source of antioxidant beta-carotene—one cup contains almost twice the RDA—as well as vitamins C and E, all of which strengthen the immune system and offer protection against heart disease and cancer. It's also a good source of fiber, calcium, and potassium. All that, along with a deep, delicious flavor that holds up well in soups and stews.

**SMART SOURCES**

*Vegetable Chronicles*, an audio series recently produced for public radio, examines the role of fruits and vegetables in preventing heart disease, cancer, diabetes, and other illnesses. It also offers tips on incorporating more produce into your meals, along with easy-to-prepare recipes and chefs' shortcuts. To order the set of four one-hour audiocassettes, call 800-554-7836.

## Kohlrabi

The marriage of a cabbage and a turnip, kohlrabi offers the advantages of both. This oft-overlooked vegetable offers 150 percent of the RDA for antioxidant vitamin C and more than 10 percent of the RDA for vitamin E. It's also rich in potassium and folic acid. Like other crucifers, kohlrabi contains anticancer compounds that help inhibit tumor formation and growth.

## Lettuce

Yes, it's 95 percent water, but don't let that fool you: lettuce is a wonderful source of nutrients. But go for the dark-leaf varieties; a whole head of iceberg won't give you the nutrition you'll find in a cup of romaine leaves. Darker leaves are especially important for their beta-carotene content; the darker the leaves, the more antioxidants they contain. Plus romaine is high in vitamin C and folic acid and contains potassium, some calcium, and a little iodine and iron. It also has antioxidant phytonutrients including flavonoids, coumarins, and lactucin.

## Mustard Greens

These dark leafy greens are as flavorful as they are healthy. Like other cruciferous vegetables, mustard greens contain indoles, compounds that help deactivate the estrogens that cause tumor growth. Plus one cup of cooked mustard greens provides almost 100 percent of the RDA for beta-carotene, 50 percent for vitamin C, and more than 10 percent for iron and calcium.

## Parsnips

Members of the *umbelliferae* family, along with carrots and celery, parsnips are nowhere near as popular—but deserve to be. Because they look like carrots drained of color, you might think they're drained of nutrients as well—but in fact these sweet and flavorful root vegetables are brimming with benefits.

Parsnips contain important cancer-fighting phytonutrients. They're also an excellent source of both soluble and insoluble fiber, and provide a good amount of folic acid, which helps prevent certain birth defects and reduces blood levels of homocysteine.

## Potatoes

Potatoes needn't be orange and sweet to be nutritious: potatoes of every persuasion are among the best foods you can eat. Among other things, white potatoes are an energizing, satisfying source of complex carbohydrates—making them, contrary to popular belief, a great choice for the weight conscious. (The only fattening part of potatoes is the butter and sour cream that are globbed on them.) A large baked potato also provides about 25 percent of your daily protein requirement; nearly half the RDA for vitamin C; nearly twice the potassium of a banana; good amounts of fiber; and B vitamins, particularly vitamin $B_6$.

## Pumpkin

Often relegated to sugary pies and Halloween jack-o'-lanterns, pumpkins should be in regular rotation as antioxidant powerhouses. Just ½ cup of canned pumpkin (which is almost as nutritious as fresh pumpkin) contains between 160 and 260

**F.Y.I.**

***Parsnips***

When you buy parsnips with the greens attached, be sure to snip off the greens before storing, or they will sap the roots of their nutrients.

To retain as many nutrients as possible, boil parsnips without peeling.

***Potatoes***

Many of potatoes' important nutrients, including potassium, are found in the skin. So try to buy organic potatoes, scrub well, and then bake rather than boil.

**F.Y.I.**

Because sea vegetables are high in sodium, it's best to use them as a flavoring or even as a garnish.

percent of the RDA for beta-carotene—that's twice as much as you'd get from the same amount of spinach. And it's a good source of other potent antioxidant carotenes, including zeaxanthin and lutein. Because these two compounds are also in the lenses of the eye, researchers believe that eating them may help prevent cataracts. Pumpkin is a good source of fiber and iron (pumpkin seeds are an even better source; see the section on nuts and seeds later in this chapter).

## Sea Vegetables

Also called seaweed, these still-exotic (in this country, anyway) vegetables are an excellent source of protein, soluble fiber, beta-carotene, folic acid, vitamin $B_{12}$—an essential nutrient many vegetarians don't get enough of—calcium, magnesium, potassium, iron, and zinc. Plus they're by far the richest food source of iodine, a mineral

### Sea Foods

These are just a few of the more popular sea vegetables:

**Kelp,** which is often used in soup and stir-fries, is rich in folic acid and magnesium.

**Kombu** has a strong flavor that stands up well in soups; it's a good source of vitamins C and A and calcium.

**Nori** is rich in protein, vitamin C, beta-carotene, and minerals. It's often used as a garnish or to wrap other ingredients, as in sushi.

**Wakame** is similar to kombu and is high in protein, iron, and calcium. It's most commonly used to make Japanese miso soup.

that's essential for normal functioning of the thyroid gland.

Considering sea vegetables' astonishing array of nutrients, it's amazing they haven't become more popular in this country—though the tide is beginning to turn. In Asia, meanwhile, they've been used for thousands of years to prevent and treat cancer and other diseases. Researchers speculate that sea vegetables contain as-yet-unidentified antioxidant compounds, some of which are not found in land plants. Their iodine content may also help prevent or treat fibrocystic breast disease, which is linked to breast cancer.

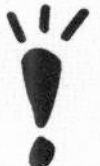

**SMART MOVE**

"Our blood contains all one hundred or so minerals and trace elements found in the ocean," notes nutritional researcher and teacher Paul Pitchford, author of *Healing with Whole Foods*.

"Seaweeds contain these in the most assimilable form because their minerals and elements are integrated into living plant tissue." Pitchford says sea vegetables contain "the greatest amount and broadest range of minerals of any organism" and are a "superb" nutritional food.

### Turnips and Turnip Greens

Another cruciferous star, the lowly turnip deserves to be put on a nutritional pedestal. Turnips contain the sulfur compound raphanol, which helps kill bacteria that cause bronchitis and other ailments. Both turnips and their big brothers, rutabagas, offer more cancer-blocking glucosinolates than other crucifers. They're a good source of vitamin C and fiber and contain small amounts of calcium, potassium, phosphorus, and some B vitamins. Turnips' green leafy tops have long been used to treat arthritis and gout because they eliminate uric acid from the body; they're also among the dark, leafy greens most often eaten by people with low rates of lung and other cancers.

GOUT + ARTHIRITIS

## Grains

The important things to remember here are *whole* grains and *complex* carbohydrates. Here's a simple rule of thumb: the more refined (i.e., processed) a grain is, the less nutrition and long-lasting energy it provides. For example, white flour and products made with it—including white bread and many other baked goods—provide very few nutrients. One caveat: there's absolutely nothing wrong with regular old pasta; even though the whole-wheat kind supplies more nutrients (and thus gets the spotlight in this chapter), pasta in any form—except drenched in fatty sauces—is a wonderful source of low-calorie, complex-carbohydrate energy.

## Buckwheat

Also known as kasha, buckwheat is not only a super source of slow-burning energy, but it also offers a multitude of healing benefits. It's rich in the flavonoid rutin, which strengthens the walls of the blood capillaries, helps prevent blood clots, maintain blood flow, and regulate fluid balance; all of which are important in preventing high blood pressure. Studies show it also helps reduce levels of damaging LDL cholesterol. Rutin and another flavonoid in buckwheat, quercetin, also appear to help prevent cancer from spreading through the body. Buckwheat eaters get an extra dose of protection from vitamin E, which combines with the grain's flavonoids to attack cancer-causing free radicals. Plus it's got zinc, copper, magnesium, and manganese.

## Bulgur

Another terrific choice for slow-release carbohydrates, bulgur, or cracked wheat, is made by soaking whole wheat in water and then baking it, which gives it a toasty, nutty flavor. Bulgur is very high in fiber and has generous amounts of potassium and

B vitamins. It also contains ferulic acid, a compound that helps prevent nitrates and nitrites in certain foods from turning into cancer-causing nitrosamines in the body. Bulgur contains antioxidant lignans, which appear to be especially effective in fighting breast and colon cancer and preventing arterial plaque.

## Millet

Like buckwheat, millet is very high in protein, making it an excellent choice for vegetarians. And because it's never highly refined, millet loses none of its essential nutrients, including magnesium, a mineral that's essential for regulating heartbeat and maintaining bone strength and nerve function; studies show it helps ease PMS symptoms as well. Millet is also rich in silicon, which is vital for healthy skin, connective tissue, teeth, eyes, hair, and nails.

## Quinoa

Quinoa is another nutrient-loaded complex carbohydrate that's extremely high in protein. And it's a complete protein, containing all nine of the essential amino acids. Quinoa is particularly rich in the amino acid lysine, which is essential for tissue growth and repair. It's also a very good source of iron: a half-cup serving provides 40 percent of the RDA for men and 27 percent of the RDA for women. Finally, quinoa provides significant doses of magnesium and riboflavin, which regulate heartbeat, maintain blood flow, and prevent dangerous clots.

## Whole-Grain Bread, Pasta, and Cereals

Rich in vitamins, minerals, and complex carbohydrates, whole wheat pastas, cereals, and whole-

**SMART SOURCES**

*It's Easy to Be Healthy with Pasta,* a brochure published by—yes—the National Pasta Association, is chock full of nutritious recipes for appetizers, soups, salads, and entrées. For a free copy, send a self-addressed, stamped envelope to:

National Pasta Association
2101 Wilson Blvd.
Suite 920
Arlington, VA 22201

grain breads are vastly superior to their refined relations. A cup of whole wheat macaroni, for example, has more than twice as much fiber as the regular kind; same for whole wheat bread. And they are good sources of antioxidant vitamin E as well. When you shop, make sure you're buying the real thing: just because the color is dark, that doesn't mean you're getting whole grain. Check the ingredient list to make sure "whole" is listed first; if it's far down the list, you may be getting only a sprinkling, and that won't do you much good.

## Dairy

As long as you avoid high-fat, high-calorie choices, dairy foods are a prime nutritional source, especially for calcium and protein.

### Eggs

Before you balk at the idea of eggs as a healthy food, take a look at what's working in their favor.

Eggs are an excellent source of high-quality protein. They provide plentiful zinc, vitamins A, D, and E, and B vitamins, especially $B_{12}$. One of their most important components is lecithin, which is vital to many of the body's metabolic processes. Lecithin helps prevent heart disease by dispersing fat deposits and cholesterol; it also helps convert fat from food into energy. And lecithin is essential for brain function: memory, concentration, and mood will all suffer if you don't get enough.

It's a mistake to avoid this nutritious, protein-rich food because of cholesterol scares. Dietary cholesterol, the kind you get from eggs and other foods, does not add to the circulating blood cholesterol and should not be a concern unless you suffer from very high cholesterol levels. Eggs are low in saturated fat, the real culprit in heart disease; studies show that saturated fat raises blood cholesterol six times as much as dietary cholesterol does. Still, researchers admit they don't yet know everything about how cholesterol works, so for the time being it's wise to keep your egg yolk consumption within the four-a-week range.

## Milk

Low-fat or skim milk doesn't have as many nutrients as the full-fat variety, but it's still a much better choice, healthwise, since the saturated fat in whole milk is far more detrimental than its nutrients are beneficial. Drinking two one-half cups of milk will give you more than the RDA for calcium—unless you're pregnant or lactating, in which case you'll get half your requirement. Milk's a great beverage choice for all women, since they are susceptible to the brittle-bone disease osteoporosis, against which calcium is a prime weapon. Calcium also helps reduce both cholesterol and blood pressure; researchers believe other substances in milk may help reduce cholesterol production as well.

Milk is also a valuable source of energy, protein, and other nutrients, including zinc, vitamin D, potassium, and riboflavin (vitamin $B_2$). These vitamins and minerals work together with calcium to keep bones healthy, making milk a much better choice than supplements. So drink up!

**SMART DEFINITION**

**Lactose intolerance**

Inability to digest cow's milk, caused by lack of a normal digestive enzyme, lactase, which is essential for the breakdown and digestion of the milk sugar, lactose.

If you experience bloating, gas, or constipation from drinking milk, you're probably lactose intolerant. But don't give up: new varieties of milk are more digestible for many people with this problem.

Many people who have trouble drinking milk find it much more digestible when consumed with food.

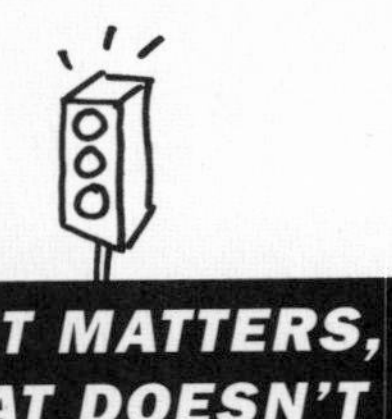

**WHAT MATTERS, WHAT DOESN'T**

**What Matters**

- Choosing meats with less than 25 to 30 percent fat.
- Eating no more than 3 to 5 ounces of meat at a meal, preferably no more than a few times a week.
- Choosing organic or free-range meats when possible to eliminate or reduce chemicals.

**What Doesn't**

- Removing all fat from meat before cooking. Trim excess fat, but don't worry about getting every bit; just be sure not to eat it.
- Avoiding red meat if you are watching your weight: a 3-ounce serving of beef tenderloin, for example, contains only 170 calories.

# Meat, Poultry, and Fish

As with dairy, you'll find an abundance of nutritional goodness in this category—but make sure you choose your proteins wisely.

## Lean Meat

Here's another much-maligned food that doesn't deserve its bad rap. Lean meat is a nutritional storehouse—in fact, it provides almost every nutrient your body needs. (But it's missing an important ingredient, fiber.) Rich in trace elements such as iodine, zinc, manganese, and selenium, meat is also an invaluable source of all the B vitamins, including thiamin (vitamin $B_1$), riboflavin ($B_2$), and niacin. Including a small amount of meat in your meal also improves iron absorption from other foods.

Pork is less fatty than beef or lamb and has little more fat than chicken if eaten without skin. But whatever meat you choose, be very careful to check the labels: all but the leanest cuts of beef can contain high percentages of saturated fat, so you can't go by the word "lean" alone.

## Chicken and Turkey

Chicken and turkey contain far less fat than other meats, and most of it is in the skin. They and other types of poultry are excellent sources of protein as well as easily absorbed iron and zinc. Poultry is rich in B vitamins: $B_6$, which is essential for making red blood cells, maintaining the nervous system, bolstering immunity, and perhaps diminishing PMS symptoms; niacin may help reduce cholesterol; and $B_{12}$ is essential for brain function—a deficiency can lead to memory loss and depression.

## Meat: The Smartest Picks

Here are the leanest, and therefore healthiest, cuts of meat to look for. All figures are for 3.5 ounces of uncooked meat:

| | Total fat (grams) | Saturated fat (grams) | Calories (grams) |
|---|---|---|---|
| **Chicken** | | | |
| Breast, without skin | 1.2 | 0.3 | 110 |
| Drumstick,without skin | 3.4 | 0.8 | 119 |
| Thigh, without skin | 3.9 | 1.0 | 119 |
| **Turkey** | | | |
| Light meat,without skin | 1.6 | 0.5 | 114 |
| Dark meat,without skin | 4.1 | 1.4 | 123 |
| **Pork** | | | |
| Tenderloin | 3.4 | 1.1 | 120 |
| Chop,top loin | 5.3 | 1.8 | 141 |
| Ham | 5.4 | 1.9 | 136 |
| **Beef** | | | |
| Top round | 2.5 | 0.8 | 120 |
| Tip round | 3.2 | 1.0 | 119 |
| Eye of round | 3.6 | 1.2 | 125 |
| Sirloin | 3.7 | 1.3 | 124 |

## Anchovies

These little fish are a big source of omega-3 fatty acids. Anchovies are also rich in the nucleic acids

**F.Y.I.**

Sulfur compounds in chicken soup help protect against infection and work to clear congestion. The so-called "Jewish penicillin" really works.

Dark poultry meat contains twice as much iron and zinc as white, but it's also higher in fat.

Meanwhile, breast meat contains double the vitamin $B_6$ of dark meat. So don't skimp on either.

Opt for free-range or organic birds when possible to avoid chemical additives.

RNA and DNA, which some researchers believe may slow the aging process by producing healthy, long-lived cells. Finally, they're a good source of vitamin A and calcium. So next time you order Caesar salad, don't tell the waiter to hold the anchovies.

## Cod

Cod and other white fish—such as haddock, catfish, snapper, sole, and halibut—are all low-calorie and are very low in fat, particularly saturated fat. White fish is loaded with protein, along with some B vitamins, iodine, and selenium. Like meat, it can also improve absorption of iron from other foods you eat at the same meal.

## Mackerel

High in beneficial omega-3 fatty acids, mackerel is one of the oily fish linked to lower risk of arteriosclerosis, arthritis, and skin diseases such as psoriasis. Omega-3 acids have also been shown to curb breast and colon cancers, reduce lung inflammation, and help women give birth to larger, healthier babies. Mackerel is a good source of vitamin D, which is essential for healthy bones.

## Sardines

Another small but mighty fish, sardines are one of the best sources of the lauded omega-3 fatty acids. They're full of protein, vitamins D and $B_{12}$, and easily absorbed iron and zinc. Canned sardines eaten with bones are an excellent calcium source.

## Shellfish

Shellfish such as shrimp and lobster contain the same amount of protein and other nutrients as white fish. Shrimp also offer niacin and copper. Mollusks—mussels, clams, and oysters—offer significantly more vitamin A and iron. Most shellfish, particularly oysters, are also a good source of zinc as well as vitamin $B_{12}$. They're also loaded with selenium, a nutrient many people don't get enough of; deficiency is linked to heart disease and greater risk of esophageal and prostate cancer. And shellfish are another good source of omega-3 fatty acids; Atlantic and Pacific oysters are especially rich in these beneficial compounds.

Most people needn't worry about the cholesterol in shellfish; in fact, high shellfish consumption has been linked to lower levels of dangerous LDL cholesterol. But if your body manufactures excess cholesterol to begin with, you should be careful not to overdo it on dietary cholesterol.

### Tuna

Meaty, rich-tasting tuna is another oily fish swimming in omega-3 fatty acids. Canned tuna is an easily accessible source of these beneficial compounds. But don't squelch all the omega-3 goodness in mayonnaise, which is rich in the wrong kind of fat.

## Nuts and Seeds

Here's another food category with a very bad—and undeserved—rap. Although high in calories, nuts are a superlative source of nutrients; eat them with salads, meat, poultry, and fish, or raw.

**F.Y.I.**

***Oily Fish***

To benefit most from omega-3 fatty acids, be sure to eat mackerel and other oily fish with foods rich in vitamin E, such as brown rice, broccoli, and asparagus. The more omega-3 you eat, the more vitamin E you need to protect the acids from oxidation, which can be harmful to your body.

***Anchovies***

To reduce their salt content, soak anchovies in a bowl of cold milk or water in the refrigerator for several hours.

***Shellfish***

Be sure to eat some vitamin C–rich foods along with shellfish in order to absorb their iron.

**F.Y.I.**

***Nuts about Nuts***

Surveys have shown that people who eat nuts—mainly almonds and walnuts—have lower rates of heart disease. In fact, eating nuts one to four times a week appears to reduce the risk of dying from heart disease by 25 percent. People who eat nuts five or more times a week may cut their risk in half. (In the American population at large, only 5 percent of people eat them that often.)

***Pumpkin Seeds***

To roast your own pumpkin seeds, first preheat the oven to 250 degrees, then clean and toss the seeds in a bowl with some olive oil until they're lightly coated. Spread in a single layer on a baking sheet, sprinkle with salt, and bake them for about an hour, or until lightly colored, turning them occasionally.

## Pumpkin Seeds

Pumpkin seeds are the richest plant source of zinc, a mineral that's essential to immune system function and for growth, wound healing, and sense of taste. It's also linked to prostate health and lower risk of bladder stones. These delicious (when roasted) seeds are also richer in iron than pumpkin flesh, with about 40 percent of the RDA for men and 27 percent of the RDA for women in a one-ounce serving—a large handful. That same amount contains 9 grams of protein, as much as in an ounce of meat. Pumpkin seeds are about 73 percent fat (most of it the good, unsaturated kind); high as that sounds, they're still lower in fat than most other seeds or nuts. They contain phosphorus, potassium, magnesium, and a huge amount of fiber (10 grams per ounce), plus a dash of vitamin A.

## Sunflower Seeds

Sunflower seeds are packed with more antioxidant vitamin E than any other common edible. Eating just an ounce of sunflower seeds a day will double most people's intake of vitamin E. They also contain large amounts of protein, B vitamins, iron, zinc, selenium, and potassium. And although they are high in fat, it's largely beneficial unsaturated fat, including linoleic acid. This fatty acid has been found to help lower cholesterol and discourage blood clots.

## Walnuts

Walnuts are another good-for-you food that have a bad-for-you rep. Although they are high in fat, it's almost all unsaturated fat and includes protective linoleic and alpha-linoleic fatty acids, the two essential fatty acids the body can't manufacture. Both have been found to help lower cholesterol and high blood pressure and prevent dangerous blood clots, as well as reduce the severity of rheumatoid arthritis and psoriasis.

Walnuts also contain ellagic acid, an antioxidant compound that appears to fight cancer on several fronts. It helps protect healthy cells from harmful free radicals, detoxifies potential cancer-causing substances, and helps prevent cancer cells from multiplying. Vitamin E, iron, selenium, and zinc round out the high nutrient profile of these nuts.

**F.Y.I.**

Although for most people chocolate is a prime feel-good food, it can make migraine sufferers feel very bad. The 20 milligrams or so of caffeine in a square of dark chocolate may be enough to launch a migraine attack.

## A Bonus Food: Chocolate

It's time to stop thinking of chocolate as sinful and start thinking of it as a food that's as good for you as it is good tasting (well, almost).

Granted, a lot of its benefits are all in your head, but still very real: One of the major ingredients of cocoa beans is theobromine, a gently stimulating chemical similar to caffeine (which is also in cocoa beans). Theobromine appears to trigger the release of feel-good endorphins in the brain—the same chemicals that kick into action when you experience love and arousal. And then there's anandamide, another cocoa ingredient that's been found to stimulate the same brain receptors as marijuana and other psychoactive drugs. In addition, chocolate's lush flavor may trigger a pleasure-induced burst of endorphins.

Though it gets more attention for its fat and sugar content, chocolate is a very good source of magnesium and iron, and it supplies protein and B vitamins as well. As for the fat, one-third of the saturated fat in cocoa butter is stearic acid, which doesn't raise cholesterol levels; another third is the beneficial unsaturated fat oleic acid.

And there's a lot to be said for a food that offers such a high return of pleasure and comfort per bite. So if you count yourself among the legion of chocoholics, come out of the closet and enjoy—in moderation.

And that's not all. . . The foods listed in this chapter and chapter 3 represent a great jumping-off point for a healthy, healing diet, but don't stop there; there's plenty more at your nearby farmstand or produce section, fish counter or natural food store. And then there's a whole world of spices and herbs, which add another layer of nutrition and pizzazz to whatever you're cooking. You'll learn more about those in the next chapter.

**THE BOTTOM LINE**

It's smart to eat the same way you live: with a sense of adventure. By including a wide range of foods in your diet, and continuing to experiment with new ones (rutabagas? papayas?), you'll be sure to get the optimum nutritional benefits nature has to offer. And you'll definitely never be bored; that may sound trivial, but in fact it's crucial to maintaining a lifelong commitment to healthy eating.

CHAPTER 5

# Healing Herbs and Spices

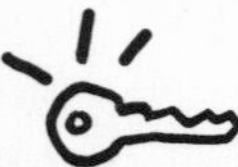

**THE KEYS**

- Condiments boost the healing quotient—and flavor— of your meals.
- Herbs and spices provide and amazing variety of health benefits.
- Try some new ideas for incorporating herbs and spices into your favorite dishes.
- Avoid pitfalls by learning the herbal dos and don'ts.
- Try out a sprinkling of healing recipes.

Herbs and spices have a long history as healing foods, one that dates back at least as far as the first century A.D., when Dioscorides wrote the first Western book on medicinal foods. But as with other foods, herbs and spices temporarily lost their healing cachet when Americans became caught up in modern technology and modern medicine. Not only that, but they lost much of their wonderful flavor as well, relegated to dusty bottles that often spent years on cabinet shelves.

Recently, however, they've enjoyed a two-part renaissance. First there was the gourmet-ization of America, as more people discovered an appreciation for fresh, flavorful foods —and in the process threw out their old condiment bottles and started growing their own herbs and purchasing spices of the best quality. Then came increased awareness and acceptance of alternative medicine, and people began looking at herbs and spices as healers.

Today Americans are catching up to most of the world's peoples, who've continued to use herbs as their primary medicine. While pharmaceutical companies spend vast amounts of money recreating the chemical makeup of herbs, more and more people are reaching for the real thing.

This chapter looks at herbs and spices that truly qualify as healing *foods*—those you can (and should) incorporate into your everyday meals both for their nourishing qualities and for their flavor. Many other herbs, such as echinacea and St. John's Wort, are used purely for medicinal purposes and are therefore not included here.

## An Important Note

Experts recommend that pregnant women avoid taking herbs; some may induce uterine contractions and induce miscarriage. Talk to your obstetrician about what's safe and what isn't.

You can find information on these and more in the recommended sources listed in this chapter.

## Herbs

What, exactly, is an herb? "The friend of physicians and the praise of cooks," said the emperor Charlemagne, and that may be as good an answer as any. Some say herbs are any "useful plants," but as James Duke, botanist and author of *The Green Pharmacy,* points out, all green plants are useful, so that doesn't help much. Duke prefers to define herbs simply as "medicinal plants."

Much research on the medicinal properties of herbs remains to be done; herbalists base many of their claims for herbs' healing powers on observation alone. However, there is increasing scientific evidence to back these claims, much of it based on research into the phytonutrients found in abundance in many of these plants.

Although many of the herbs listed below may prove beneficial when taken in medicinal doses—and most offer little risk of side effects—you should only do so on the recommendation of your health practitioner. But incorporating herbs in your healing menus is a guaranteed route to boosting nutrition and flavor.

### Basil

Among the most popular of herbs, basil has a sweet flavor that marries well with all sorts of Italian dishes.

Basil contains monoterpenes, phytonutrients with disease-fighting antioxidant properties. It aids digestion and can soothe cramps, upset stomachs, and gas,

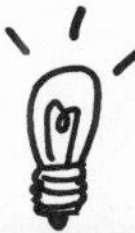

**STREET SMARTS**

***Basil Tea***

"I make basil tea after big meals, or after eating foods that don't agree with me—most of which I still can't resist," says Laurie Berg, twenty-nine, a public relations executive. "It not only calms my stomach but also soothes me all over. Sometimes it soothes me so much I fall asleep!" She steeps 2 teaspoons of dried basil in 1 cup boiling water for 15 minutes, then strains.

***Storing Basil***

To enjoy basil year-round, blend fresh leaves with enough olive oil to make a smooth paste. Then freeze in an ice cube tray and add to soups or pasta all winter long.

You can also chop basil or other herbs, put 1 tablespoon per cube in an ice cube tray, add water, store in a heavy plastic bag, and freeze.

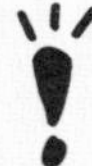

**SMART MOVE**

"Herbal remedies are a safe and healthy alternative to sleeping pills," notes Richard Craze, a stress management consultant and author of *Herbal Teas*. "They are nonaddictive and gentle." The most commonly used, and probably most effective, sleep-aiding herb is chamomile, according to Craze, who recommends a cup of chamomile tea before bed.

To make this or other herbal teas, steep 1 or 2 teaspoons of dried herb in 1 cup of hot water for 5 minutes. Then strain and drink.

perhaps thanks to a compound called eugenol, which has been shown to ease muscle spasms. It also acts as an antiseptic and a mild sedative.

**Try it in . . .** dishes containing pasta, tomatoes, chicken, fish, shellfish, and eggs; basil is most famously used in pesto, a pasta topping made with ground pine nuts, olive oil, garlic, and Parmesan cheese.

## Bay Leaf

This aromatic, deep-flavored seasoning is an antiseptic and a mild stimulant. It stimulates digestive juices and improves absorption of nutrients from food; it also helps prevent gas and cramps. Bay leaf contains phytonutrients called parthenolides that may help prevent migraine headaches. Parthenolides inhibit release of serotonin from blood platelets; researchers believe that serotonin release plays a role in causing migraines.

USDA research also has shown that bay leaf helps the body use insulin more efficiently and can help stabilize blood sugar levels, making this a useful herb for diabetics.

**Try it in . . .** hearty bean soups and stews.

## Chamomile

Best known as a calming herb, chamomile is often used to make teas that treat insomnia and jangled nerves. It also contains anti-inflammatory compounds that can help ease arthritis.

Chamomile is a traditional cure for menstrual pain and tension as well as pregnancy-related sickness. Chamomile also has antiseptic properties and can help fight bacterial and fungal infections.

**Try it as . . .** an herbal tea.

## Chives

Chives have a light onion flavor and share many healing properties of garlic and onions, which belong to the same allium family. Like their brethren, they have antibacterial and antiseptic properties, and research indicates they may help prevent cancer and reduce high blood pressure. Their smell and taste also improve the appetite and stimulate digestive juices.

**Try them in . . .** dishes containing fish, shellfish, or eggs; they're also great in soups and salads.

**F.Y.I.**

Add fresh herbs such as chives and cilantro to dishes right before serving to preserve their full flavor and nutrients.

## Coriander/Cilantro/Chinese Parsley

The nutty seeds and clean-tasting leaves (some call them "soapy," which is a rather unappetizing description for this popular herb) of this plant are essential in Mexican, Latin American, and Asian cooking.

Coriander contains antioxidant flavonoids as well as the essential oils linalol, pinene, and terpinine, which help soothe the digestive system and have antiseptic, antibacterial, and antifungal properties.

**Try it in** . . . dishes containing rice, beans, fish, or shellfish; salads; salsas.

## Dill

Dill is available both as seeds and herb (often called dillweed). The seeds are more intensely flavored and are spices used to make pickles, and in rice and fish dishes; the leaves are milder and used in egg, seafood, vegetables and poultry dishes.

Dill contains antioxidant volatile oils such as carvone and limonene that help relieve stomach pain, heartburn, and other digestive problems.

**F.Y.I.**

Allicin is formed when garlic is cut or crushed. If the aroma is destroyed, as in cooking, garlic no longer acts as a microbe killer, though it may still have other healing properties.

**Try it in . . .** potato, tomato, and cucumber salads, as well as the above-mentioned dishes.

## Fennel Seeds

The licorice-like flavor of fennel is particularly popular in Mediterranean fish recipes. The plant's active ingredients are most concentrated in its seeds, which contain the volatile oils anethole and fenechone, as well as antioxidant flavonoids.

Fennel seeds help ease intestinal cramps and upset stomach and improve digestion. They also have an estrogen-like effect, helping to stimulate menstruation and the production of breast milk, as well as ease the symptoms of menopause.

**Try it in . . .** bouillabaisse, salmon dishes, tea.

## Garlic

The most famous of all healing foods, garlic has a healing reputation that dates back thousands of years. An ancient Egyptian papyrus listed some twenty-two garlic-based remedies, and the list hasn't shrunk since then. Among other benefits, garlic has been reputed to lower blood pressure; lower the risk of heart disease, stroke, and cancer; improve circulation; and lower blood sugar levels. It also has antibacterial and immunity-building properties.

Allicin, the compound that gives garlic (and onions) its strong odor, is an antibiotic that may be more powerful than penicillin and tetracycline. It works even against such powerful disease-spreading microbes as tuberculosis and botulism, along with more common infections such as colds, flu, stomach viruses, and yeast infections.

Lab studies have shown that another compound found in garlic, diallyl sulfide, inactivates potential cancer-causing substances and prevents tumor growth. Garlic compounds also stimulate production of the amino acid glutathione, a potent antioxidant. Researchers believe garlic's antioxidant powers may be even stronger than those of vitamin E.

Garlic not only kills bacteria but also stimulates the immune system, which helps the body fight infectious diseases—and possibly cancer and AIDS as well. It also thins the blood, helping to prevent dangerous blood clots, and lowers blood pressure.

One thing garlic may *not* do, however—despite myriad reports to the contrary—is lower blood cholesterol levels. New research indicates that garlic clove supplements have no effect on cholesterol. Still, further tests need to be done before the results are conclusive.

**Try it in . . .** just about anything—except desserts!

## Lemon Balm

With its sweet and tangy taste, lemon balm makes a great addition to summer salads and soups. The volatile oil citronella and other flavonoids help calm the nerves and treat mild depression; some researchers believe it can help treat migraine. Lemon balm also has antiseptic and antibacterial properties that help soothe indigestion.

**Try it in . . .** fruit salads, tea.

## Licorice

The root of the licorice plant is a powerful healing herb. Licorice contains glycyrrhizic acid, a phytonutrient fifty times sweeter than sugar that acts as a potent anti-inflammatory and also as an

**F.Y.I.**

Licorice sold as candy in the U.S. is usually flavored with anise, so don't eat it for its healing benefits. The European version, however, often has a high licorice content.

antibiotic against the bacteria that cause cavities. (Licorice components are often used in mouthwash.)

Licorice root also contains striterpenoids and phenolics, compounds that may help prevent cancer. Licorice is a traditional ulcer treatment as well.

**Try it in . . .** tea.

## Mint

There are more than thirty varieties of this herb, all of them blessed with a refreshingly cool flavor and smell.

Mint contains the essential oils menthol, menthone, menthyl acetate, and flavonoids, which have antiseptic properties and soothe sore throat, toothache, and digestive problems. Mint also helps relieve headaches, especially stress headaches. The antioxidant monoterpenes in mint may also prevent cancer and heart disease.

**Try it in . . .** tabbouleh; bean, potato, or fruit salad; tea.

## Oregano

It's hard to find a Mediterranean or Mexican dish that doesn't contain this much-loved herb, which marries well with many foods.

Oregano may have more antioxidant properties than any other herb, which means it's a potent weapon against the free radical damage that can cause premature aging, cancer, heart disease, and other woes. Its essential oil has antiseptic properties and is useful in treating respiratory and digestive problems.

**Try it in . . .** fish, chicken, egg, bean, and vegetable dishes and tomato sauces.

## Parsley

The most widely used culinary herb, parsley may also be the most underrated healing food. Don't make the mistake of using parsley merely as a decorative garnish. If it's served to you that way, don't leave it sitting on the plate—eat it!

Parsley is loaded with vitamin C and beta-carotene—ten sprigs provide 15 percent of the RDA for C, and 10 percent for beta-carotene. It's also rich in iron, calcium, folic acid, and potassium.

Parsley contains other active substances as well, including polyacetylenes, which block synthesis of prostaglandins that may promote cancer; coumarins, which help prevent blood clotting and are also believed to have anticancer properties; flavonoids, antioxidants that also help prevent tumor growth; and monoterpenes, antioxidants that help reduce cholesterol.

**Try it in . . .** bean soups, tomato sauces, salads, and poultry and fish dishes.

**SMART DEFINITION**

**Volatile oil**

An oil that vaporizes easily and that gives a plant its characteristic smell and flavor (e.g., citronella in lemon balm and rosemaricine in rosemary).

## Rosemary

Rosemary's strong piney aroma and flavor come from the volatile oil rosemaricine along with other compounds such as camphor, limonene, and flavonoids. It fortifies the immune system, strengthens blood vessels and improves circulation, stimulates digestion, and increases urine flow, helping to rid the body of harmful toxins. Rosemary also contains antioxidant compounds called quinones that have been shown to fight cancer-causing toxins.

Rosemary is called the herb of "remembrance," and lives up to its reputation. Its compounds increase blood flow to the head and stim-

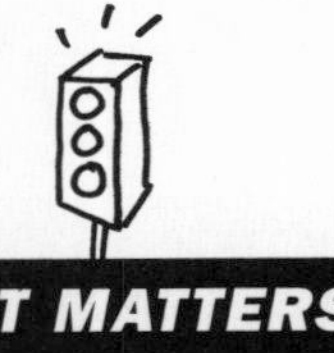

**WHAT MATTERS, WHAT DOESN'T**

**What Matters**

- Using fresh herbs whenever possible to maintain optimal flavor and nutrients.
- Adding herbs to dishes just before serving.

**What Doesn't**

- Measuring fresh herbs precisely; using a little more than a recipe calls for won't hurt the dish—and will boost its health quotient.
- Sticking to the classics—try substituting different fresh herbs in your favorite recipes.

ulate the brain's cortex, improving concentration and memory; this also soothes nerves and tension headaches and helps improve mood.

**Try it in . . .** chicken, turkey, and meat dishes; also roasted potatoes, mushrooms, and melon (yes, melon).

## Sage

Musky-flavored sage was dubbed the "immortality herb" by the ancient Greeks, and it does indeed promote long, if not eternal, life. Sage contains the volatile oil thujone, bitters, flavonoids, and phenolic acids, which have antioxidant, antiseptic, and anti-inflammatory properties and aid digestion. Thujone is also a phytoestrogen and helps relieve menstrual pain and menopause symptoms.

Researchers have recently discovered that sage may be a useful weapon against Alzheimer's disease. Its compounds inhibit the enzyme that breaks down acetylcholine, a compound that appears to help prevent and treat the disease.

**Try it in . . .** soups and stews; poultry or eggplant dishes.

## Thyme

A pungent, minty herb, thyme contains volatile oils that may act as antioxidants and have antiseptic properties that strengthen the immune system against viral, bacterial, and fungal infections. Thyme is particularly useful against stomach viruses and yeast infections. The essential oil thymol is used to make antiseptics and mouthwashes.

**Try it in . . .** poultry, fish, and shellfish dishes; also goes well with tomatoes, beans, potatoes, and mushrooms.

## Spices

Spices come from the seeds, roots, fruits, buds, or bark of plants. (Herbs generally, though not always, come from the leaves.) They're a wonderful kitchen staple because they retain their full flavor and healing properties when dried, and they remain potent for many months when stored airtight.

**F.Y.I.**

In the nineteenth century, women carried cardamom seeds in their pockets—an early version of breath fresheners.

### Anise

These small seeds taste like licorice and contain the essential oils anethole and estragol, which aid digestion and help clear congestion. In large doses, anise may also have antiviral properties.

**Try it in . . .** tea.

### Caraway

Caraway seeds have a nutty flavor similar to licorice and are commonly used in Europe as a digestive aid. They contain the compounds carvone, limonene, and pinene, which soothe stomach pains and act as gentle diuretics. Caraway also helps relieve congestion and soothes coughs.

**Try it in . . .** dishes containing cabbage, potatoes, beets, or turnips; egg dishes.

### Cardamom

Cardamom is a warming, cinnamon-like spice that helps relieve digestive problems such as indigestion, vomiting, diarrhea; and stimulates the appetite. It also contains cineole, a compound that helps reduce congestion and phlegm, as well as antibiotic compounds that help fight tooth decay. Cardamom tea may help relieve anxiety.

**F.Y.I.**

Clove oil is a top toothache remedy around the world.

**Try it in . . .** curries and other Indian foods; also dishes containing sweet potatoes and winter squash. It's a great addition to traditional rice pudding.

## Cayenne

For benefits, see chili peppers in chapter 3.

**Try it in . . .** egg dishes and vegetable dips.

## Cinnamon

This popular spice gets its hot, sweet flavor from the volatile oil cinnamaldehyde, which is one of the strongest natural antiseptics; it can help prevent and treat everything from colds to chronic infections. Eugenol in the oil acts as a painkiller and a mild sedative; it helps relieve muscle and joint pain, headaches, and toothache, and also helps lower blood pressure. Compounds called catechins make cinnamon an effective weapon against nausea and indigestion. It has also been shown to help control blood sugar levels.

**Try it in . . .** applesauce; also in dishes containing carrots, sweet potatoes, or winter squash.

## Cloves

The most stimulating aromatic spice, cloves have a pungent flavor that warms the body, revs up circulation and digestion, and relieves nausea. They contain the compound eugenol, a very effective blood thinner, as well as compounds that have antiviral, antibacterial, and antifungal properties. Their tannins also help relieve diarrhea.

**Try it in . . .** dishes containing sweet potatoes, winter squash, or carrots.

## Ginger

Warm, spicy ginger is most famous as an effective treatment for nausea and motion sickness. But its healing powers extend much further than that. Ginger contains zingeberene, gingerols, and shogaols, compounds that lower cholesterol and blood pressure; may reduce heart disease and cancer risk; help prevent blood clots (ginger is a more powerful anticoagulant than either garlic or onions); relieve migraine headache; and improve circulation.

Researchers have found that both fresh and dried ginger have healing benefits, but dried ginger is much more potent than fresh.

**Try it in . . .** stir-fries and other Asian fare; stewed fruit; and tea.

**F.Y.I.**

Just ½ teaspoon of dried ginger, or a small piece of fresh or candied ginger, will help treat motion sickness.

## Horseradish

A relative of watercress, horseradish shares many of its healing benefits. Its isothiocyanantes provide strong antibiotic, antibacterial, and anticancer properties. Horseradish is also rich in sulfur, which aids digestion and clears congestion; just a spoonful will do the trick.

**Try it in . . .** soups and vegetable dips;and in condiments for roast meats and grilled fish.

## Juniper

These strong-flavored dried berries contain a compound called deoxypodophyllotoxin that has been shown to inhibit herpes and flu viruses, among others. They also aid digestion and are a traditional treatment for urinary tract infections.

**Try it in . . .** marinades for meat, poultry, and fish.

**SMART SOURCES**

You'll find detailed information on both culinary and medicinal herbs and spices in the following books:

*The Encyclopedia of Medicinal Plants* by Andrew Chevallier

*The Healing Kitchen: An Indoor Herb-Garden Pharmacy for Cooks* by Patricia Stapley

## Mustard

Zesty mustard seeds have potent antimicrobial and anti-inflammatory properties and stimulate the immune and digestive systems. Dry mustard provides good amounts of magnesium, which helps the body manufacture protein, build bones, and metabolize other nutrients.

**Try it in . . .** spice mixtures to rub on poultry and fish before cooking; salad dressings.

## Mace and Nutmeg

Mace is the lacy outer covering of nutmeg; both spices are sweet and nutty. Nutmeg and mace help stimulate the appetite, improve digestion, and relieve nausea thanks to myristicin, a compound that is chemically similar to mescaline (from the peyote cactus in Mexico).

**Try them in . . .** dishes containing broccoli, onions, carrots, cauliflower, or Brussels sprouts; eggnog; also with fruits such as peaches, plums, and apples.

## Saffron

This brilliant-colored spice is made from the stigma of crocuses and is as expensive as it is flavorful. Just a tiny bit adds deep flavor to Spanish dishes.

Saffron contains crocetin, a chemical that has been shown to lower blood pressure. Some researchers link the low heart disease rate among Spaniards to high saffron consumption.

**Try it in . . .** paella, bouillabaisse, risotto, and other seafood dishes.

### Turmeric

A relative of ginger, this bright yellow spice is potently flavored and essential to mustards, curry powder, and relishes.

One compound in turmeric, called curcumin, acts like aspirin to inhibit the synthesis of prostaglandins, the chemicals that make us experience pain. Turmeric also contains phytonutrients that may help prevent cancer, according to the National Institute of Nutrition in India—the country with the highest per capita turmeric consumption by far.

**Try it in . . .** Indian curries and rice dishes.

## The Big Picture

Although culinary herbs and spices offer myriad benefits in and of themselves, they are also crucial to the bigger dietary picture. When you flavor dishes with them instead of the old standbys such as rich sauces, butter, and excess salt, you open up whole new vistas of healthy eating.

***THE BOTTOM LINE***

Herbs and spices are essential ingredients in any healthy kitchen, not only because they are brimming with healing properties, but also—and just as importantly—because their extraordinary flavor makes every good-for-you dish a great-tasting one as well. And that is no small thing; what you are eating may be "good medicine," but it certainly should not taste that way!

CHAPTER 6

# The Food Doctor

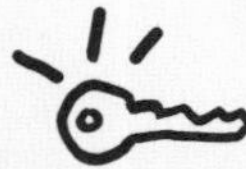

**THE KEYS**

- Disease and diet: how what you eat determines the way you feel.
- Browse an alphabet of common ailments: their causes, symptoms, and treatment.
- For each ailment, learn the nutrients you need, and why.
- There are specific foods to prevent and treat each disease.

The key to preventing disease is taking care of yourself. That means eating a wide assortment of the foods recommended in this book, as well as other foods rich in nutrients and fiber and low in saturated fat and empty calories. It also means limiting your alcohol intake, avoiding other drugs (including nicotine), and maintaining a healthy weight and active lifestyle. All pretty simple stuff.

Unfortunately, there's nothing simple about disease—its causes are complex and still largely unknown. Although eating smart is essential for good health, it doesn't *guarantee* good health.

If you have a medical condition or recurrent health problem, dietary changes may lessen or prevent its recurrence. But food is not a cure-all. If you are being treated for a specific medical problem, don't make any changes in your treatment plan without consulting your health practitioner.

# An A-to-Z of Ailments

The following are nutritional recommendations for a variety of ailments, from minor to major.

## Acne

A common skin disorder among teenagers, acne also plagues some adults, particularly those with oily skin. Its cause is not completely understood, but in adolescence it is probably linked to hormonal changes that affect the skin's oil glands and ducts, which produce sebum, a skin lubricant.

Overproduction of sebum can cause blockage in hair follicles, which can lead to inflammation and, in turn, pimples.

Keeping your skin clean is one very important factor in controlling acne. Another is diet. Contrary to popular myth, eating potato chips one day will not lead to a breakout the next; but it's no myth that eating a diet high in fat and low in nutrients can only do bad things for your skin. Fiber, zinc, vitamins A and E, and essential fatty acids are all especially helpful.

***Smart Foods***

- Shellfish, salmon and other oily fish; lean meat for zinc.
- Apricots, carrots, and yams for beta-carotene.
- Wheat germ and walnuts for vitamin E and essential fatty acids.

## Anemia

When you have insufficient red blood cells or hemoglobin in your blood, less oxygen reaches your body's tissues. That can lead to the tiredness, weakness, dizzy spells, irritability, and depression associated with anemia.

Anemia is most often caused by heavy bleeding through menstruation or other causes, or by lack of essential nutrients—mainly iron, but also folic acid, vitamins $B_6$ and $B_{12}$, vitamin C, as well as protein—required to make red blood cells. It most frequently affects teenage girls and pregnant women.

***Smart Foods***

- Oily fish, dried beans and peas, pumpkin seeds, leafy green vegetables, parsley, apricots, wheat germ, and fortified cereals and breads for iron and folic acid.

## Iron Overload

Too much iron can be as bad as too little. Excess iron can interfere with the body's absorption of zinc, which is essential for the immune system; it may also cause oxidative damage to the cells (acting as an anti-antioxidant), which can lead to cancer and other serious illnesses. Talk to your health practitioner before taking iron supplements.

- Citrus fruits, red peppers, watercress, and other leafy green vegetables for vitamin C.
- Brussels sprouts and other cruciferous vegetables, avocados, and bananas for vitamin $B_6$.
- Lean meat and sea vegetables for vitamin $B_{12}$.

## Arthritis

There are two basic types of arthritis, both of which cause swelling and pain in the joints. In osteoarthritis, joint cartilage hardens or erodes and causes bone spurs and lumps. In rheumatoid arthritis, joints become inflamed, causing soreness and stiffness.

Although there are as yet no cures for arthritis, many experts believe eating certain foods may help prevent or minimize arthritis pain; for example, omega-3 fatty acids have been found effective in alleviating symptoms. Avoiding other foods, including members of the nightshade family—potatoes, tomatoes, and eggplant—may also help.

***Smart Foods***

- Oily fish, such as salmon and mackerel, for omega-3s.
- Chili peppers and pineapple to help relieve inflammation.
- Apples, celery, and parsley to help reduce swelling.
- Fresh ginger may help too, according to some studies, by blocking inflammatory substances.

## Asthma

Asthma is triggered by foreign substances that enter the body and inflame bronchial passages. Stress can worsen attacks; eating right can help minimize them.

Foods rich in omega-3 fatty acids and the antioxidants vitamins C and E and selenium help the body fight inflammation and respiratory diseases, and battle free radicals generated by air pollutants in the lungs. Vitamin E, along with the mineral magnesium, also helps smooth airway muscles in the lungs, making breathing easier.

***Smart Foods***

- Oily fish such as sardines and salmon.
- Citrus and other fruits and vegetables rich in vitamin C, such as mangoes, red peppers, and Brussels sprouts.
- Wheat germ and almonds for vitamin E.
- For selenium: chicken, seafood, lean meat, and—the very best source—Brazil nuts.
- Onions, to help prevent bronchial constriction.
- Tea, which contains theophylline, a compound that's been shown to dilate the bronchial tubes.

## Cancer

Cancer has become the most dreaded word in the English language. The fear stems not only from its deadly reputation (it's the second most common cause of death in the United States) but also from the notion that there's no way to prevent it. In fact, however, there's more and more evidence that you can greatly reduce—if not eliminate—your risk of cancer, simply by opting for a healthy diet and an active lifestyle.

The term cancer refers to more than a hun-

**SMART DEFINITION**

**Types of Cancer:**

**Carcinoma** is cancer that affects the skin, mucous membranes, organs, and glands.

**Leukemia** is cancer of the blood.

**Sarcomas** are cancers of the muscles, connective tissues, and bones.

**Lymphoma** is cancer of the lymphatic system.

**SMART SOURCES**

According to the National Cancer Institute, the nearly fifteen thousand chemical additives that help preserve, flavor, and color foods are "subjected to extremely careful laboratory screening before they are used, and scientists believe it is unlikely that they contribute significantly to the overall cancer risk in humans." If you have questions about specific food additives, contact:

U.S. Food and Drug Administration
Center for Food Safety and Applied Nutrition
Direct Additives Branch
200 C St. SW
Washington, DC 20204

dred diseases involving abnormal growth of cells within organs or tissues. The tumors formed by these cells can be either benign or malignant. Benign tumors, the nondeadly kind, do not spread to surrounding tissue; cells from malignant tumors do, often causing tumors in other parts of the body.

Cancer starts when the unstable oxygen molecules called free radicals damage healthy cells and prevent normal cell activity and growth. Researchers link the preponderance of cancers to various factors, including diet, smoking, stress, sexual and reproductive history, and occupational hazards. Chemical pollutants and environmental conditions are other major suspects.

According to the National Cancer Institute, there is no evidence that any kind of diet, food, or vitamin or mineral supplement can either cure cancer or stop it from coming back; however, there is much evidence that certain foods can help prevent cancer from happening at all. Foods that are low in fat, and high in fiber and antioxidant nutrients—including vitamins C and E and beta-carotene, selenium, and phytonutrients—are your best cancer-preventive prescription.

***Smart Foods***

- All the foods in this book!

## Cataracts

The leading cause of eyesight loss among elderly Americans, cataracts result from proteins that accumulate inside the eyes' lenses and from degeneration of the macula, the part of the retina responsible for visual detail. Many factors may contribute to cataract formation, but good eating habits—particularly early in life—can help reduce their occurrence. Particularly important are antioxidant vitamins beta-carotene, C, and E, as well as the B vitamin riboflavin, which seems to help prevent cataract formation.

***Smart Foods***

- Spinach, broccoli, carrots, apricots, and pumpkin for beta-carotene.
- Citrus fruits, cantaloupe, mangoes, papayas, kale and other leafy green vegetables, and other foods rich in vitamin C.
- Sunflower seeds, wheat germ, and avocados for vitamin E.
- Chicken, eggs, mushrooms, low-fat milk and yogurt, and wheat germ for riboflavin.

## Colds and Flu

Although there's still no cure for the common cold, a strong immune system is the key to fighting off such viral infections and minimizing their duration. Fruits and vegetables provide the best immunity-building arsenal; make sure you get at least the USDA's recommended "five a day"—preferably more.

Once you're in the grips of a full-blown cold or flu, you can eat certain foods to relieve congestion and other symptoms. But touted cold treatments, such as megadoses of vitamin C or zinc, will not zap a virus from your system; at best, they may help shorten the duration of a cold or flu by a few days. The best medicine is preventive: stock up on virus-fighting nutrients all year long, not just during cold and flu season.

***Smart Foods***

- Fruits and vegetables rich in antioxidant vitamins and compounds, such as citrus fruit, broccoli, leafy greens, and red peppers.

**SMART SOURCES**

Major cancer research organizations offer a wealth of information about eating smart to help prevent and treat cancer.

The American Institute for Cancer Research publishes a booklet called *From Around the World: Menus and Recipes to Lower Cancer Risk,* filled with ideas for tempting, nourishing meals. For a free copy, send a self-addressed stamped envelope (55 cents postage) to:

American Institute for Cancer Research
1759 R St. NW
Washington, DC 20009

The National Cancer Institute's *Action Guide to Healthy Eating* offers tips on building your resistance and disease-fighting power through good nutrition. It's available online at:

rex.nci.nih.gov/nci_pub

**F.Y.I.**

When food starches and sugars break down into glucose in the blood, the pancreas produces the hormone insulin, which enables glucose to leave the bloodstream and enter cells, where it is used as energy or stored. People with diabetes don't produce insulin, produce too little, or produce enough but become unable to use it (known as insulin resistance). Their cells are deprived of energy, which causes weakness, dizziness, and a variety of other health problems, including poor circulation.

Worse still, glucose can become toxic when it sits in the bloodstream for too long, damaging your organs. The link between diabetes and cardiovascular disease is acutely direct: some 80 percent of diabetes sufferers eventually die of heart or blood vessel disease, according to the American Heart Association.

• Garlic, onion, and watercress, to fight infection and bronchial congestion.
• Chili peppers and ginger to relieve congestion, stimulate circulation, and soothe the stomach.
• Honey to soothe the throat.
• Tea and homemade chicken soup to relieve congestion and boost immunity.

## Constipation

Keep two words in mind when it comes to constipation: fiber and fluids.

Constipation is usually a sign that you are eating too many of the wrong things—processed, refined foods—and too few of the right ones: fruits, vegetables, whole grains, and legumes. It also may mean you aren't drinking enough water and other healthy fluids, or that you are drinking too much alcohol and coffee, which can cause dehydration. (In moderate amounts, however, coffee stimulates the digestive tract and can help relieve constipation.)

Both fiber and fluids are essential to help your body move food through your digestive tract and eliminate waste. When you don't eat right, you not only throw your digestive system out of whack, but you also increase your risk of certain cancers, such as colon cancer, because your body is not eliminating potentially dangerous toxins as efficiently as it should.

***Smart Foods***

• Prunes, apricots, apples, bananas, and cruciferous vegetables such as broccoli for fiber and fluid.
• Lentils and dried beans, oats, and other whole grains for fiber.
• Water, to keep the fiber moving through your body.

## Diabetes

There are two types of diabetes: in Type I, or insulin-dependent diabetes, the body manufactures little or no insulin. Type I sufferers, who include children and young adults, often require insulin injections throughout their lives. Researchers don't yet know what causes this type of diabetes, but there is a tendency to inherit it.

Type II diabetes, or insulin-resistant diabetes, is much more common, particularly among inactive, overweight people over 40. These people produce some insulin, but not enough. Diet is both a direct cause and treatment for this form of diabetes; the best prescription is often improved eating and exercise, which often enables Type II diabetics to use more of their own insulin and balance their blood sugar with diet alone.

Both types of diabetes can be controlled by eating foods high in fiber and complex carbohydrates, which cause a minimal rise in blood sugar levels; avoiding excess refined sugar; and eating frequent small meals. It's also important to consume enough vitamin $B_6$, chromium, zinc, and magnesium; diabetics often have low levels of all four.

***Smart Foods***

- Apples, bananas, dried beans, wheat germ, and other foods high in soluble fiber help stabilize blood sugar levels.
- Whole-grain bread and cereal, pasta, corn, dried beans, and fruits and vegetables for complex carbohydrates.
- Turkey, fish, walnuts, potatoes, avocados, red peppers, broccoli and other cruciferous vegetables for vitamin $B_6$.
- Lean meat, shellfish, dried beans and peas, nuts,

**SMART SOURCES**

The National Diabetes Information Clearinghouse puts out a number of informative, reader-friendly publications, including *Diabetes Dateline,* a quarterly newsletter; *The Diabetes Dictionary,* an illustrated glossary of more than 350 diabetes-related terms; and several booklets addressing the needs of diabetes patients. All are available online at:

www.niddk.nih.gov/health/diabetes/ndic/htm

**F.Y.I.**

Diarrhea hits everyone occasionally; usually contaminated food or drinking water is to blame, but it can also stem from incomplete digestion or overuse of antacids or laxatives. If you are afflicted with chronic diarrhea, however, you may have a more dangerous intestinal condition that requires medical attention. See your physician for an evaluation.

whole grains, and pumpkin seeds for chromium and zinc.
• Shrimp, wheat germ, tofu and other soy foods, dried apricots, brown rice, and nuts and seeds for magnesium.

## Diarrhea

Diarrhea is characterized by frequent and liquid bowl movements that can cause dehydration, weakness, nausea, gas, abdominal pain and cramps, and sometimes fever and vomiting, not to mention inconvenience.

It's impossible to avoid occasional bouts of diarrhea, but eating the right foods can help prevent some cases and can help shorten its duration. If you have lactose intolerance, for example, eating milk and other dairy products may cause diarrhea and other digestive problems. Overconsumption of fruit can also cause trouble for some people.

***Smart Foods***
• Water and fruit juices to replenish fluids, sugars, and minerals that are depleted by diarrhea.
• Bland foods such as brown rice, bananas, and whole-grain bread to soothe the digestive tract and provide fibrous bulk.
• Wine, which may kill diarrhea-causing bacteria.

## Gout

Gout, a close relative of arthritis, was long associated with aristocrats who enjoyed a diet rich in fatty foods and alcohol; nowadays it affects millions of people—primarily overweight men over forty, but postmenopausal women, too. It's caused by an excess of uric acid in the blood, which leads to crystallized deposits that cause joint pain and swelling, particularly in the big toe. That may sound like a minor affliction unless you've experienced it; the inflammation can be excruciating.

Gout is a hereditary disease, but poor metabolism, an aristocratic diet high in fat and alcohol, and excess pounds increase your risk of developing it. So far, there's no cure, but medication is often effective, and eliminating certain foods from your diet can help prevent it. Experts recommend avoiding excess alcohol; it's also a good idea to eat fewer foods that are high in purines, substances that the body converts into uric acid. These include organ meats such as liver; fish such as anchovies, sardines, and mackerel; and vegetables such as asparagus, and legumes.

***Smart Foods***

- Water, to dilute uric acid in the bloodstream and help prevent crystallized deposits.
- Celery and celery seed, which also help eliminate uric acid.
- Turmeric, which helps reduce inflammation and pain.

## Headache

The list of headache-makers is a long one: stress, noise, tiredness, weather, and hormonal changes are all common causes, as are some of the foods we eat and the liquids we do or don't drink.

Whatever the cause, the result is one of two types of head pain: tension headaches, which are caused by muscle contraction in the neck and scalp, and vascular headaches, including the often excruciatingly painful migraines, which are caused by expansion and contraction of blood vessels in the head and neck.

When it comes to headaches, what you *don't* con-

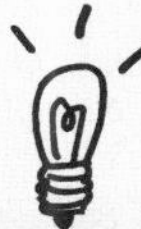

**STREET SMARTS**

Jeri Wray, a fifty-one-year-old receptionist and grandmother who has suffered from migraines since age eighteen, says she has sworn off caffeine and wine, two foods that tend to trigger her headaches. And she's careful about other potential problem foods as well. "Maybe two or three times a year I'll have a bit of chocolate, but that's it," she says. "Instead of getting on the medication merry-go-round, which can cause rebound headaches on its own, I'm much more into trying to avoid things that give me migraines, and living healthy."

## Headache Triggers

The following are just a few of the foods that have been linked to headaches, particularly migraines; if you are susceptible, you may want to try cutting these from your diet for a while to see if it makes a difference:

- Nitrates from smoked meats, hot dogs, and other preserved foods, which cause blood vessels to dilate, causing throbbing head pain.
- Chocolate, aged Cheddar and other cheeses, and red wine; they contain the amino acid tyramine, which can also make blood vessels contract and dilate.
- MSG (monosodium glutamate), most commonly found in Chinese food but also in canned soups and other prepared foods, which causes headaches in many people, though researchers aren't yet sure why.

sume can be as important as what you do. Unfortunately, there's no easy way to tell whether your headaches are food-related, or which foods they may be related to, but if you are a frequent headache sufferer it's worth making the extra effort to pinpoint food culprits. Keeping a headache diary will help: keep track of when you get your headaches and what you ate in the preceding twenty-four hours; over time you may be able to pinpoint the problem foods.

But it's not all about eliminating foods from your diet; there are also certain nutrients you should get in order to help prevent headaches. Calcium, iron, and magnesium are effective against head pain, particularly the headaches associated with PMS. And vitamin $B_6$ is helpful for coping with stress, a common headache trigger.

***Smart Foods***

- Low-fat yogurt and milk, tofu, leafy green vegetables, and almonds for calcium.
- Lean red meat and potatoes for iron.
- Wheat germ, whole grains, nuts and seeds, bananas, apricots, and shrimp for magnesium.
- Wheat germ, walnuts, fish, turkey, bananas, and potatoes for vitamin $B_6$.

## Heart Disease

Heart attack is the number one killer of Americans; stroke is number three—and the number one cause of debilitation. Both come courtesy of heart disease.

After studying heart disease for decades, researchers have a pretty clear picture of what makes it happen and what you can do to help prevent it. When arteries become clogged by plaque, they can't carry sufficient oxygen-bearing blood to the heart. That leads to heart disease. Heart attacks happen when the heart's arterial passageways are completely blocked by plaque or by blood clots; stroke happens when the brain's arteries are similarly blocked.

Some of the risk factors for heart disease are out of your control: age, gender (men are at greater risk than women, and they have attacks earlier in life), and heredity. Others, however, are well within your control. Aside from smoking and inactivity, all the other risk factors cited by the American Heart Association involve diet.

The dietary keys to heart health are eating foods that are low in saturated fat and high in antioxidant vitamins, particularly vitamin E and beta-carotene, as well as potassium, which regulates blood pressure. Eating foods high in omega-3 fatty acids have also been shown to have a heart-healthy effect.

***Smart Foods***

- Wheat germ, sunflower seeds, almonds, sweet potatoes, broccoli, and leafy green vegetables for vitamin E.
- Red peppers, apricots, mangoes, pumpkin, carrots, and leafy green vegetables for beta-carotene.
- Dried fruit, leafy green vegetables, potatoes, bananas, and citrus fruit for potassium.

**SMART SOURCES**

The American Heart Association publishes numerous free pamphlets on nutrition and heart disease, including *The American Heart Association Diet, Cholesterol and Your Heart,* and *Facts About Potassium,* along with publications on exercise and other crucial lifestyle factors. For more information, call the AHA at 800-AHA-USA1 or check out the AHA Web site at: www.americanheart.org

**F.Y.I.**

High blood pressure is caused by several factors. High cholesterol levels cause arterial plaque buildup and atherosclerosis (narrowing and hardening of the arteries), which make it harder for your heart to pump blood through your body. Being overweight is another major risk factor: the more pounds you carry, the harder your heart has to work to pump blood to your tissues. Excess sodium is also directly linked to elevated blood pressure in many people.

• Salmon, sardines, anchovies, and other oily fish for omega-3 fatty acids.

## Hemorrhoids

Hemorrhoids are varicose veins that develop near the anus and rectum. Heredity can make you more prone to hemorrhoids, and chronic constipation, obesity, and poor circulation most certainly increase your risk. Hemorrhoids can also occur during pregnancy, when there's lots of pressure on veins. As with constipation, the most frequent culprit is a diet high in processed foods and fat and low in fiber and fluids.

***Smart Foods***
• Whole grains, legumes, bananas, apples, and other fruits and vegetables for fiber.
• Ginger and garlic to stimulate circulation.
• Blueberries and cherries for proanthocyanidins, which help strengthen vein walls and capillaries.
• Water (at least six to eight glasses a day) to keep fiber moving through the body.

## High Blood Pressure

Eating right can have a dramatic effect on your blood pressure—and that's no small matter, considering that high blood pressure is very closely linked to heart disease and stroke risk.

Avoiding saturated fat and salty foods, if you are sensitive to sodium, can help lower blood pressure. So can increasing your intake of fiber, potassium, and calcium.

***Smart Foods***
• Sweet and white potatoes, parsley, celery, fennel, leafy green vegetables, and dried apricots for potassium, which helps regulate sodium.

• Lowfat yogurt and milk, tofu, canned fish with bones, and watercress and other leafy greens for calcium.
• Fresh herbs and spices, vinegar, and lemon juice to replace salt as seasoning.

## Kidney Stones

The kidneys dispose of waste products from the blood and thus are temporary home to excess minerals and other substances. Kidney stones form when some of these waste products—usually calcium oxalates, but also uric acid or phosphates—crystallize and form hard lumps. When these get lodged in the urinary tract, the pain can be excruciating; some have compared it to childbirth or worse. Unfortunately, kidney stones are usually not a one-time event; if you haven't had them yet, it's wise to do what you can to prevent them.

***Smart Foods***
• Wheat germ, whole grains, soy foods, shrimp, and dried apricots for magnesium.
• Potatoes, bananas, citrus fruits, and dried fruit for potassium.
• Water (at least six to eight glasses a day) to keep your body well hydrated.

## Osteoporosis

Loss of bone minerals causes osteoporosis—porous bones that fracture easily and heal poorly.

Unfortunately, the mineral most important to bone health, calcium, is the one most likely to be absent from low-fat diets that exclude dairy foods such as milk and cheese. Older women are especially vulnerable to brittle, weakened bones because as their estrogen levels begin to decline (around age forty), so does their ability to absorb

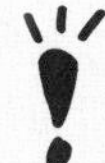

**SMART MOVE**

James A. Duke, Ph.D., author of *The Green Pharmacy* and a world-renowned expert on plants and natural healing, believes doctors are "too quick to treat high blood pressure with synthetic drugs" and asserts, "There's plenty of solid evidence that...diet and lifestyle changes, including regular exercise, stress management, and self-monitoring with a home blood pressure device, work just as well as drugs, with no side effects."

Duke recommends regular doses of vegetable soup: "It's so good for health I don't call it minestrone anymore, but rather Medistrone." There's no precise recipe for Medistrone, but it always includes heart-healthy ingredients such as garlic, onions, red pepper, ginger, and tomatoes; other antioxidant-rich vegetables; and cholesterol-lowering beans.

**SMART SOURCES**

For more information about kidney stones and other urologic diseases, check out the National Institute of Diabetes and Digestive and Kidney Diseases Web site at www.niddk.nih.gov/

calcium. Both women and men use vitamin D less efficiently as they age, which also appears to reduce calcium absorption.

Although osteoporosis is not a problem for young people, consuming sufficient amounts of calcium, vitamin D, and other bone-strengthening nutrients, such as boron and phytoestrogens, at an early age is essential to maintaining bone health later.

***Smart Foods***

- Lowfat yogurt and milk, tofu, sardines, and other canned fish with their bones, almonds, and leafy green vegetables for calcium.
- Lowfat milk, salmon, mackerel, and other oily fish for vitamin D.
- Apricots, prunes, and other dried fruit for boron.
- Soy foods, dried beans, and whole wheat breads and cereals for phytoestrogens.

## Psoriasis

This scaly red skin condition results when skin cells reproduce too quickly; it most often afflicts the scalp, elbows, legs, and knees, but it can occur on other body parts. Researchers don't yet know what causes psoriasis, but it tends to be inherited and often is linked to arthritis.

Although there's no known cure for psoriasis, studies have shown that a low-fat, nutrient-rich diet helps alleviate the condition. Avoid saturated fats in particular, and seek out beneficial omega-3 fatty acids, which are in low supply among many psoriasis sufferers. Omega-3s appear to inhibit inflammation, which can trigger psoriasis. It's also important to get vitamin D, the "sunshine" vitamin, by spending time outdoors and by eating foods rich in this nutrient. Finally, be sure to eat plenty of antioxidant-rich produce to keep your immune and digestive systems in peak form.

***Smart Foods***

- Salmon, sardines, and other oily fish for omega-3 fatty acids and vitamin D.
- Tomatoes, carrots, and other vegetables and fruits rich in vitamins C, E, and beta-carotene.
- Garlic, ginger, and hot peppers to improve circulation.

## Stroke

Stroke occurs when blood stops reaching parts of the brain. High cholesterol and high blood pressure, both of which can interfere with blood flow, greatly increase your risk of stroke. Therefore, it's crucial to closely monitor your intake of saturated fat, which raises cholesterol levels leading to clogged arteries in the heart, and maybe in the brain—which in turn leads to stroke. Obesity is a major cause of high blood pressure, so watch your weight.

Eat foods high in fiber and antioxidant nutrients, as well as potassium, which has been shown to lower blood pressure and reduces your risk of developing blood clots. Foods rich in B vitamins, particularly $B_6$, $B_{12}$, and folic acid, help regulate levels of the amino acid homocysteine, which has been linked to heart disease and stroke risk.

***Smart Foods***

- All fruits and vegetables, as well as whole grains, for fiber.
- Apricots and other dried fruits, bananas, leafy green vegetables, and potatoes for potassium.
- Wheat germ, spinach, watercress, parsley, legumes, and orange juice for folate.

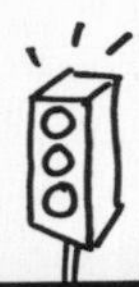

**WHAT MATTERS, WHAT DOESN'T**

### What Matters

- Eating regular meals that are rich in high-fiber foods.
- Avoiding iron supplements; iron is a gastric irritant.
- Avoiding caffeine and alcohol while you have an ulcer.

### What Doesn't

- Avoiding spicy foods; it's a myth that bland diets prevent or treat ulcers.
- Drinking milk to "coat" the stomach; too much milk can encourage harmful acid production.
- Avoiding stress so that you won't develop ulcers; most experts believe stress does not cause ulcers, but it *can* exacerbate existing ones.

- Turkey, fish, sweet red peppers, Brussels sprouts, and other cruciferous vegetables for vitamin $B_6$.
- Chicken, extra-lean meats, and sea vegetables for vitamin $B_{12}$.
- Tea, which contains flavonoids that have been shown to greatly reduce stroke risk.

## Tooth Decay

Of the three essentials for preventing tooth decay, two are well known: brushing and flossing regularly, and avoiding sugary snacks. The third is equally important, although often overlooked: eating foods that will keep your teeth strong and resistant to attack from harmful acids.

Calcium-rich foods are essential for healthy teeth, building strong teeth when you are young, and maintaining bones that hold your adult teeth in place. Vitamin A is essential to form dentin, the bonelike layer beneath teeth's surface; vitamin C is important in preventing oral infections.

***Smart Foods***

- Lowfat yogurt and milk, tofu, sardines and other canned fish with their bones, almonds, and leafy green vegetables for calcium.
- Mangoes, cantaloupe, carrots, and red peppers for vitamin A.
- Tomatoes, leafy green vegetables, citrus fruit, and potatoes for vitamin C.
- Tea, which contains polyphenols and tannins that act as antibiotics and kill bacteria, as well as tooth-protective fluoride.
- Cheese—a small cube at the end of a meal appears to reduce risk of tooth decay, possibly by neutralizing acids before they can cause damage.

## Ulcers

Ulcers are open sores that form in the digestive tract, causing inflammation and pain. They are caused by a breakdown in the mucous lining that protects the stomach from the damaging effects of stomach acid.

Caffeine, alcohol, and heavy meals all overstimulate acid production and can be troublesome for those people prone to ulcers. Good guys include soluble fiber, which may help stop ulcers from returning; zinc, which helps heal ulcerous sores; and foods with strong antibacterial properties, such as yogurt.

***Smart Foods***

- Fruits, vegetables, whole grains, and beans for fiber.
- Lowfat yogurt with live *Lactobacillus acidophilus* cultures to kill harmful bacteria.
- Sunflower and pumpkin seeds, shellfish, and whole wheat bread for zinc.
- Raw cabbage and cabbage juice; cabbage contains the amino acid glutamine, which increases blood flow to the stomach and helps strengthen its lining.
- Raw, unpasteurized honey; it strengthens the stomach lining and helps kill ulcer-causing bacteria.

**F.Y.I.**

You may inherit a susceptibility to ulcers; other causes include bacterial infection and adverse reactions to food and medications. Aspirin and other anti-inflammatory drugs attack the mucous lining. Surprisingly antacids can spell trouble too, by triggering a rebound rise in acid.

And more important: Bleeding ulcers can be life-threatening. Of course, if you spit up blood, contact your doctor immediately.

## Yeast Infections

Most women harbor the *Candida albicans* fungus, which causes vaginal yeast infections and the itching and discomfort that accompanies them. But the fungus doesn't cause trouble unless your immune system allows it to get out of control. Taking antibiotics can kill the beneficial bacteria that halt fungal growth; other medicines, including oral contraceptives, may also help the bacteria to flourish.

***Smart Foods***

- Nonfat and lowfat yogurt with live *Lactobacillus acidophilus* cultures, which has been shown to lower yeast infections in women who consumed 8 ounces a day.
- Garlic, which has been shown to kill the fungus in lab tests; results are still preliminary.

**THE BOTTOM LINE**

Sound nutrition is the foundation for good health and disease prevention. In many cases, eating the right foods can also help treat illness. In others, diet and physician-prescribed medicines and treatment can work together to speed your recovery. But remember that food and medications work in different ways; while you can pop a pill for immediate relief, good eating is a lifetime prescription.

# Index

# Books in the **Smart Guide**™ Series

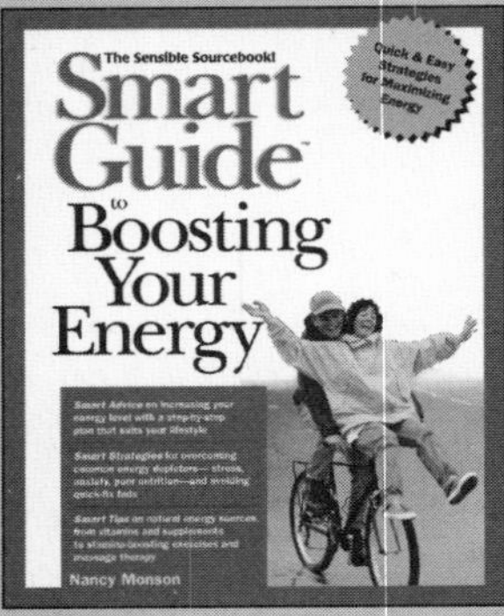


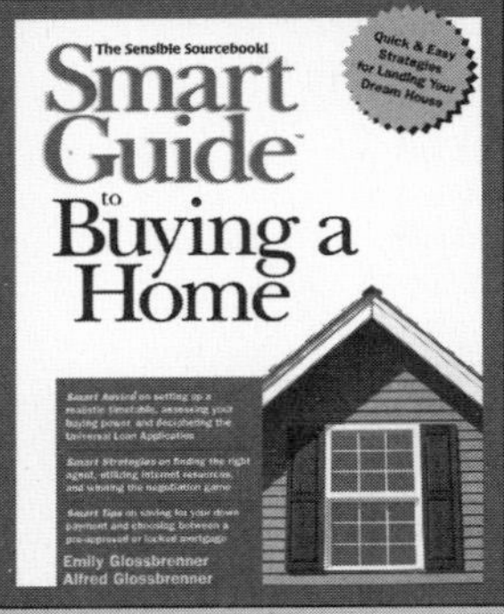


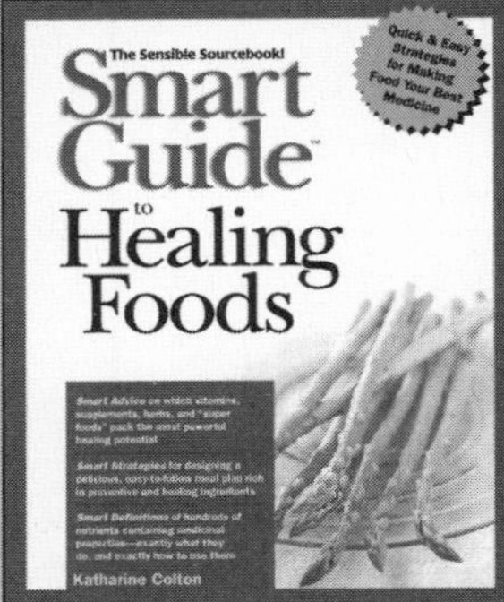


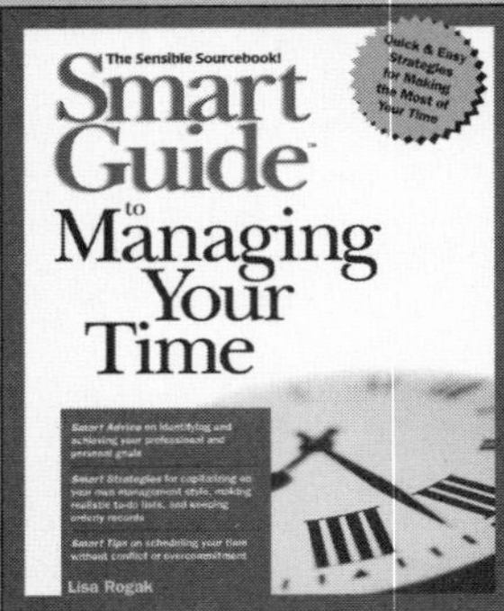


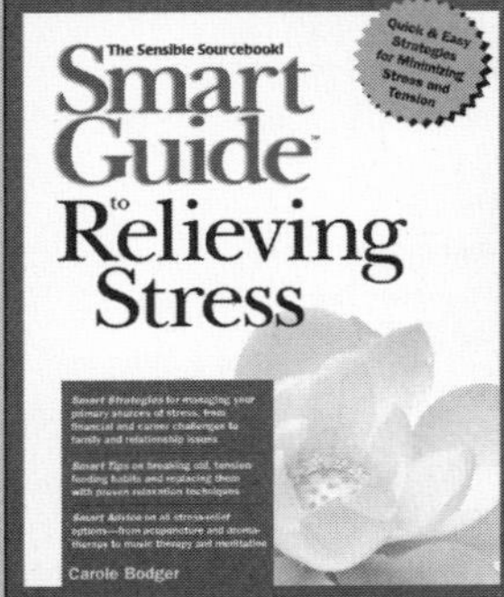


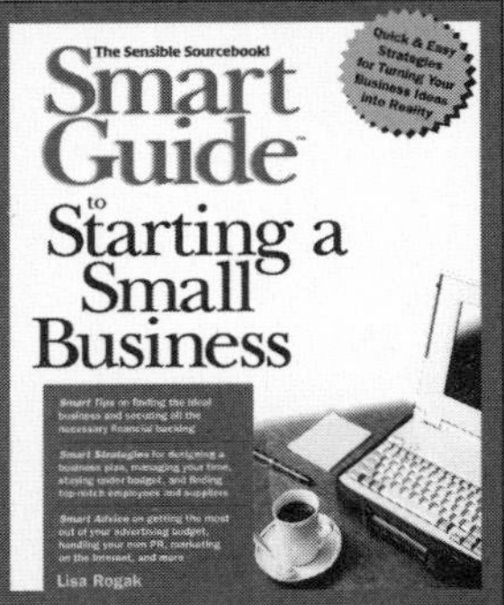


Smart Guide™ to Boosting Your Energy

Smart Guide™ to Buying a Home

Smart Guide™ to Getting Strong and Fit

Smart Guide™ to Getting Thin and Healthy

Smart Guide™ to Healing Foods

Smart Guide™ to Making Wise Investments

Smart Guide™ to Managing Personal Finance

Smart Guide™ to Managing Your Time

Smart Guide™ to Profiting from Mutual Funds

Smart Guide™ to Relieving Stress

Smart Guide™ to Starting a Small Business

Smart Guide™ to Vitamins and Healing Supplements

**Available soon:**

Smart Guide™ to Healing Back Pain

Smart Guide™ to Maximizing Your 401(k) Plan

Smart Guide™ to Planning for Retirement

Smart Guide™ to Planning Your Estate

Smart Guide™ to Sports Medicine

Smart Guide™ to Yoga